WHAT (ALMOST) NOBODY WILL TELL YOU ABOUT SEX

a student journal

jim hancock & kara eckmann powell

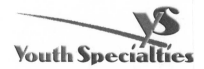

Youth Specialties

D1451066

ZondervanPublishingHouse
Grand Rapids, Michigan

A Division of HarperCollinsPublishers

What (Almost) Nobody Will Tell You about Sex: A student journal

Copyright © 2001 by Jim Hancock and Kara Eckmann Powell

Youth Specialties Books, 300 S. Pierce St., El Cajon, CA 92020, are published by Zondervan Publishing House, 5300 Patterson Ave. S.E., Grand Rapids, MI 49530.

Library of Congress Cataloging-In-Publication Data

Hancock, Jim, 1952-
    What (almost) nobody will tell you about sex : a student journal / Jim Hancock
& Kara Eckmann Powell.
      p. cm.
   ISBN 0-310-23716-5
    1. Sexual instruction—Religious aspects—Christianity. 2. Sex instruction for
youth. 2. Sexual ethics for youth—Study and teaching. 4. Church work with
youth. I. Powell, Kara Eckmann, 1970- II. Title.

HQ59 .H36 2001
241'.66'0712—dc21

00-043881

Edited by Tamara Rice, Lorna McFarland Hartman, and Dave Urbanski
Cover design and interior photography by Proxy
Interior design by Razdezignz

Printed in the United States of America

01 02 03 04 05 06 07 / / 10 9 8 7 6 5 4 3 2

CONTENTS

It doesn't take a genius to know that everything we hear about sex can't be true. Some people say sex is a purely natural and biological urge, so knock yourself out—don't look for any meaning. Other people say sex is an almost sacramental act of communication between a man and a woman committed for life.

Gimme a break. How's anybody supposed to figure out the truth?

Almost no one expects an honest, well-thought-out answer from the church. Your church is probably very cool on the issue of sex, but most seem to have lost their voices on the subject. Some churches are speechless because they're just as confused and afraid about sex as everybody else. Other churches scream themselves hoarse defending positions that aren't necessarily all that clear in the Bible. And parents—not yours, of course, but most—are about as helpful as most churches. Some are just scared silent. Others have talked so much they have laryngitis. In either case, we see their lips moving, but it's hard to make out what they're saying. So a lot of us stopped listening.

Wouldn't it be nice to have a reasonable, direct, honest, genuine, hopeful conversation about sex? Wouldn't it be great to talk about God's gift of sex in optimistic—but not unrealistic—terms? Wouldn't it be wonderful to mention sex without fear or anger or pretending? Or waiting for the lecture that's sure to follow?

Well, it would be nice, and it's entirely possible. Not easy, maybe, but entirely possible. That's why we wrote this book.

Here are some of the big ideas behind *What (Almost) Nobody Will Tell You about Sex:*

- We're created in God's image, male and female.

- Sexuality is a wonderful, complex gift that takes a lifetime to explore.

- Sex touches every part of us. Our bodies, sure. But also our minds, emotions, spirits, and every relationship—with our families, with the God who makes us, and with everyone else.

- Sex is affected by our brokenness and wrongdoing, just like everything else about us.

- Sex can be rescued and renewed by the grace of Christ, just like everything else about us.

What (Almost) Nobody Will Tell You about Sex is designed to help you understand sex in the broad context of your whole life.

If our strategy is to look at sex in the context of the whole person, our tactics involve a collection of self-contained-but-still-connected elements—bite-sized experiences to get you thinking and talking and deciding what you will do with God's gift of sex.

What (Almost) Nobody Will Tell You about Sex is organized into seven chapters.

- **SexTalk**—responding to the cultural messages you're wading through
- **Sexual Identity**—thinking about the forces that shape your sexuality
- **Intimacy**—dating and nonsexual closeness
- **Desire**—understanding your appetites and needs
- **Boundaries**—deciding how to conduct yourself sexually
- **Do-Overs**—experiencing mercy, repentance, forgiveness, and restoration

(We've also added The Stuff at the Back of the Book: Plumbing and Wiring—FAQs, Back-to-Basics Biology, How to Help Victims of Sexual Abuse, and All the Sex in the Bible.)

Each chapter includes an essay and a collection of questions to think about, write about, and maybe even talk about. Look for three elements as you read.

GOD'S-EYE VIEW provides you with a biblical perspective on the topic.

THINK ABOUT IT allows you to reflect on the issues and questions listed.

WRITE ABOUT IT invites you to journal your thoughts, emotions, and ideas.

There's a logic to the order of *What (Almost) Nobody Will Tell You about Sex,* but don't let the table of contents slow you down. If you feel the need to jump straight to **Do-Overs** because you or a friend needs a fresh start, then do it (as if you needed our permission). You don't have to wait until you understand everything—which may never happen—to share the truth of God's forgiveness with those who know they really need it.

In the real world, we encounter sexual information and experiences in a process that stretches over decades. And out of that process—or in the middle of it—we construct our ideas and values about sex. Most of that information, and quite a bit of that experience, is indirect. We read books and magazines and Web pages. We listen to the radio. We watch television and movies. We hang out with siblings, friends, and acquaintances. We watch our parents and other adults. We experience sexual arousal, and it takes us by surprise!

From these impressions, we construct a picture of what sex is or appears to be. And from that picture come our sexual attitudes, opinions, and actions. The picture is updated each time we encounter new information and experiences, and even in adulthood the picture is never complete as long as we're learning.

Take a moment to compare that process of learning about sex with most teaching about sex. Most of what kids get directly from adults is much less a process and much more a confrontation: "Here are the facts—remember them. This is the truth—believe it. These are the boundaries—don't cross them." But we've made **What (Almost) Nobody Will Tell You about Sex** more of a process than a confrontation because that's how people really learn.

Once we reach puberty, we're always talking about relationships with the other gender. We're exposed to films, books, magazines, music, and television shows that constantly talk about sex, dating, love, and marriage (often in that order). We live in a human context that's often, on one level or another, about sex. It's all part of the process. Except at church (and a few other adult-sensitive settings), where grownups confront instead of process. Come to think of it, that *is* part of the process, whether it's a conscious choice or not. That's one reason kids grow up believing it's not safe to talk about sex when adults are around.

Let's just get this out on the table. What the Bible says about sexuality goes against almost everything else we hear on the subject. Our culture, our bodies—every fiber of our being—screams for sex early and often. But early and often isn't exactly a biblical approach to responsible, intimate, disciplined, pleasurable, committed, passionate sex. So we're in a bit of a bind. Either our culture and our bodies are right about sexual fulfillment, and God just forgot to mention it—or God is perfectly clear about the sexual experiences that are most fulfilling, useful, helpful, and ultimately pleasurable, and we just have a tough time understanding how to get there.

An ancient Hebrew ritual celebrates a fascinating process of leading children into loving obedience to their invisible Creator:

> Hear, O Israel: The Lord our God, The Lord is one. Love the Lord your God with all your heart and with all your soul and with all your strength. These commandments I give you today are to be upon your hearts. Impress them on your children. Talk about them when you sit at home and when you walk along the road, when you lie down and when you get up. Tie them as symbols on your hands and bind them on your foreheads. Write them on the doorframes of your houses and on your gates.
>
> —Deuteronomy 6:4-9

Now *that's* process. Sitting around the house, walking around the block, bedtime stories and morning devotions, a bracelet on your arm, a do-rag on your head—all day, every day, thinking about what God wants. People who get that wrapped up in what God wants tend to do what God wants, in the same way that people who get wrapped up in what they want tend to do what they want. Funny how that process works.
Here's another idea from the Bible.

> Do not conform any longer to the pattern of this world, but be transformed by the renewing of your mind. Then you will be able to test and approve what God's will is—his good, pleasing and perfect will.
>
> —Romans 12:2

What (Almost) Nobody Will Tell You about Sex is a process between you and God (and maybe a few people you really trust). It's an invitation to go deep into the process of being transformed by God.

We also created a package for youth groups called **Good Sex**. It's a resource that invites whole groups to consider, understand, and surrender their sexuality to the God who loves them and made them sexual. The youth group package covers everything in *What (Almost) Nobody Will Tell You about Sex* (plus a bunch more) and invites group interaction and support. Your youth group leader can get **Good Sex** curriculum by calling 800-776-8008 or by visiting a Christian bookseller.

This book won't answer every one of your questions about sex. How could it? Instead, it's loaded with great questions to help you wrestle with God's truth and your own experience.

And that's the combination that makes the difference—God's truth shaping your experience.

SexTalk

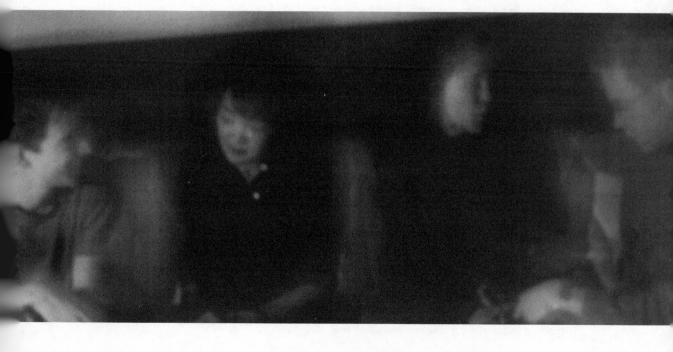

SEXTALK

Suppose you came to a country where you could fill a theatre by simply bringing a covered plate onto the stage and then slowly lifting the cover so as to let everyone see, just before the lights went out, that it contained a mutton chop or a bit of bacon, would you not think that in that country something had gone wrong with the appetite for food?
—C. S. Lewis, *Mere Christianity* (Macmillan)

Something has gone wrong with our appetite for sex. No matter how you look at it, our cultural fascination with sex is out of proportion to its actual significance. That may be hard to see because nothing has changed in your lifetime.

You've grown up pretty much unprotected from what grownups cynically refer to as *adult content*. You never knew a world without home video and cable sex, explicit language on pop radio, or one-click access to Internet material that might have gotten your grandfather kicked out of the house (maybe even thrown in jail).

You also never knew a world without HIV/AIDS and rampant outbreaks of sexually transmitted diseases—a world where careless sex can sterilize or even kill.

What can we say that's useful in the world where you actually live as opposed to Never-Neverland where things are the way they're supposed to be? Should biblical thinkers throw up their hands or dig in their heels? Should they ignore biblical messages written "too long ago and too far away" to be much use in the 21st century? Alter them to fit modern sensibilities? Or hunker down and defend their tiny square of turf until the last one dies off and the world goes to hell?

Oddly enough, what the Bible says about sex may be more helpful today than ever. Most everybody agrees we're in a mess. We're sexually confused and no one seems to be doing much about it. Of course, almost nobody wants to go back to pretending people don't think about sex until their wedding night. No one looks at the era of sneaky sex and believes people were more noble then because they lied about their behavior. And who in their right mind wants to go back into hiding about sexual abuse and leave women and children vulnerable to assault?

Most people assume the Bible is hopelessly out of touch about modern sex. It's not. The Bible's message flourished in times when acceptable sexual behavior was far more abusive than ours. Those folk lived in cultures in which male and female prostitution was part of religious life (so just imagine life among the pagans). They lived in towns where sacrificing girls was the main event at the shrine on the hill. They lived in cities where boys were sex objects for wealthy men. They lived in cultures where women were property—collected, traded, used, and discarded. And no one raised an eyebrow, let alone a helping hand.

> You don't change the old by resisting it but by replacing it with a superior technology.
> —Buckminster Fuller, 20th-century inventor and social critic

The people of God blew into those cultures like a fresh, but very strange, breeze. They brought hope and a wind of change. And not so much by their words as by their lives.

God's people reinvented the family by introducing committed marriage, instilling respect for women, and protecting and nurturing children instead of exploiting them.

These ideas were huge, not because smart people wrote about them, but because ordinary people lived them out. Think of what we know about sexual abuse—most abusers were themselves victims of abuse when they were young. There's every reason to believe it's always been that way. Which means that adult believers who were abused as children chose to break the cycle of abuse—they chose to give better than they got. Adult believers chose to treat their wives as partners instead of property. Adult believers who grew up one way chose another way to live by the power of God's Spirit—so children weren't disposable, marriages weren't temporary, and sex wasn't violent. That was world-changing stuff.

Maybe it's time to do that again. Because somehow the people of God lost the thread of sexual wholeness. We talk like we know what's going on, but no one listens anymore, because our actions speak louder than words.

So maybe it's time to stop talking and, quietly but steadily, help each other grow into our sexuality healthy and whole. We can do that with God's grace—not because we're good, but because God is so very good. Maybe it's time for us to give better than we got. It's within our reach.

where did you learn about sex?

WRITE ABOUT IT

Q: The following activity will help you think about where you've learned about sex. What have you learned about sex from these sources, and how true to life do you think the information is?

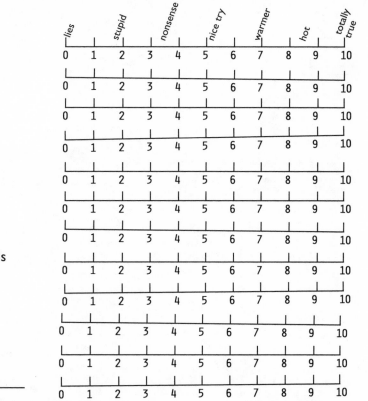

- romance novels
- music
- sex ed
- soap operas
- movies
- visual porn
- locker room talk
- sleepover gossip and confessionals
- parent-child sex talks
- youth group talks
- Christian books and speakers
- Other: _____

Scale for each: lies (0 1) stupid (2 3) nonsense (3 4) nice try (4 5) warmer (5 6) hot (7 8) totally true (9 10)

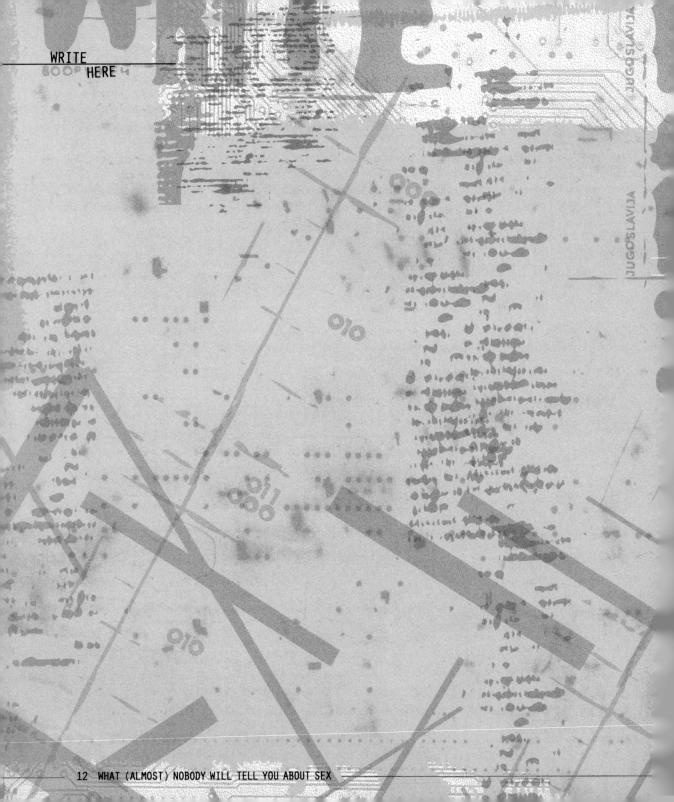

Q: How reliable does your information about sex seem to be so far?

Q: Have you gotten hurt by any bad info?
- Do you think there's any difference in the reliability of sources for boys and girls? Why?

Q: Where do you wish you had learned about sex?
- If someone came to you for advice on where to learn about sex, where would you send that person? Why?
- What do you think the Bible says about sex? (If you're not quite sure, we think you will be by the end of this book.)

> I wish someone had told me about the mechanical parts that just aren't very sexy at all—just the mechanics of making everything fit right.
>
> —Brian, on being prepared for his wedding night

where in the world are you?

WRITE ABOUT IT

Circle the percentage that describes how each statement applies to you.

0% means it's not true at all for you today.	50% means it's half true for you today.	100% means it's completely true for you today.

- I have very little interest in sex.   (0%) ——— 50% ——— 100%

- I think about sex, but I don't do anything about it.   0% ——— 50% ——— (100%)

- I fool around a little.   0% ——— (50%) ——— 100%

- I fool around a lot.   (0%) ——— 50% ——— 100%

- I've had sex.   (0%) ——— 50% ——— 100%

- I've been molested.   (0%) ——— 50% ——— (100%)

- I've been forced to have sex or raped.   (0%) ——— 50% ——— 100%

- I'm having sex in the relationship I'm in now, but I'm careful.   (0%) ——— 50% ——— 100%

- I've been having sex for a while and with a number of partners. I'm always very careful.   (0%) ——— 50% ——— 100%

- I used to have sex more than I do now.   (0%) ——— 50% ——— 100%

- I'm not sexually active right now, but that could change if the right person came along.   0% ——— 50% ——— (100%)

- I've been tested for sexually transmitted diseases since the last time I had sex.   (0%) ——— 50% ——— 100%

The last time I had sex was—

❑ in the last week.
❑ in the last month.
❑ in the last three months.
❑ in the last six months.
❑ in the last year.

❑ in the last two years.
❑ in the last three years.
❑ more than three years ago.
☒ never.

Q: Look over your answers. If you didn't know who filled out this form, what do you think you could learn about that person by reading these responses?

girls, guys, and changing bodies

THINK ABOUT IT

Q: In general do you think our culture places more value on how we look on the outside or who we are on the inside? Why do you think that?
   • What do you think God would say about this? What makes you think that?

Q: What physical qualities does our culture value in women? How are those values communicated?

Q: What physical qualities does our culture value in men? How are those values communicated?

Q: Do you think the pressures to look a certain way are greater for women than for men? Why do you believe that?

WRITE ABOUT IT

Q: Does that sound about right to you?
   • Why do you think boys became less unhappy with their bodies by age 18?
   • Why do you think girls became more unhappy with their bodies by age 18?
   • Do you think there's anything that can be done about girls' dissatisfaction? Why?

Q: Regardless of whether you're a girl or a guy, how does all this impact your own life?

> In February 1999, the Henry J. Kaiser Family Foundation released a study indicating that two-thirds of prime-time TV shows and 56 percent of all TV shows include sexual content. The shows with the most sex are soap operas, movies, and talk shows. According to this study, relatively few of these shows offer "responsible" sexual messages about contraceptive use, abstinence, or protection from sexually transmitted diseases.
>   These findings prompted Health and Human Services Secretary Donna E. Shalala to compare TV sex to the distorted mirror at a carnival fun house.
> —*Cheryl Wetzstein*, Washington Times (September 13, 1999)

> Lots of girls who are trying to lose weight are fighting against their very biology.

> In a study of 117 subjects at ages 13, 15, and 18, overall body dissatisfaction emerged between ages 13 and 15 and was maintained at age 18. While boys became less unhappy with their bodies, girls became more unhappy with their bodies.
> —*Gianine Denise Rosenblum*, "Body Image, Physical Attractiveness and Psychopathology During Adolescence," doctoral dissertation, Rutgers University

write here

pick one

Circle your answer.

Do you think sex seems—

thrilling or scary
fun or painful
better for men or better for women
complicated or simple
more physical or more spiritual
more mental or more emotional

GOD'S-EYE VIEW

I don't know about you, but I'm tired of pretending sex has to be one thing or the other. The reality is that sex is all of the things you just voted on. Under the right circumstances, sex is fun and relaxing. Under the wrong circumstances, sex is scary—maybe even painful. Sex can be 100 percent right, and it can be 100 percent wrong.

But for now, let's focus on the last two statements: sex is more physical or more spiritual, and sex is more mental or more emotional.

Sex is physical—there's no doubt about that. But I believe sex is more than just physical. I believe sex relates to what we think, how we feel, and how we relate to God and to each other. Trying to choose whether sex is more physical, spiritual, mental, or emotional is a bit like asking whether a human being is more physical, spiritual, mental, or emotional—we're all of them, all the time.

Q: If you had a girlfriend/boyfriend/husband/wife, and the two of you got all your information from magazines or novels, what percentage of your life together do you think would be devoted to each part—mental, physical, spiritual, and emotional?

% mental

% physical

% spiritual

% emotional
_____

100 %

• Do you believe those percentages can support healthy relationships between healthy people? Why or why not

WRITE HERE

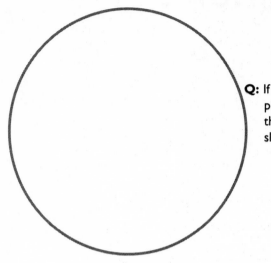

Q: If your experiences with sex so far were in the shape of a pie, how big would the physical slice be? How about the intellectual slice? Emotional? Spiritual? Try drawing the slices on the circle to the left.

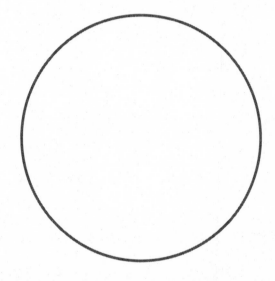

Q: What do you think is the *ideal* size of each slice? Try drawing them in the circle to the right.

Q: When you compare the circles, what does this tell you about how you view sex?

GOD'S-EYE VIEW

The reality is that God designed you as a whole person—what happens in your brain affects what happens in your heart, which affects how you relate to God and other people, which ultimately affects what you do with your sex organs. It seems to work in the other direction too. What a woman does with her sex organs affects what goes on emotionally, relationally, intellectually, and spiritually. What a man does with his sex organs affects what goes on emotionally, relationally, intellectually, and spiritually. Maybe it's not this clear and simple, but it's entirely possible that your sexuality is more wrapped up in who you are mentally, emotionally, spiritually, and socially than you've been led to believe by our culture.

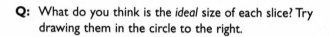

Your primary sex organ is not between your legs but between your ears.

Q: If that's true, what two or three things could you do to keep these areas in balance?

sexual sanctuary

Q: If you have a youth group, is it a safe place to discuss the whole truth and nothing but the truth about sex?

> Sex is both one of the most overrated and underrated experiences. The media makes such a big hype about sex, focusing almost solely on the physical aspects, as if good sex can solve all your problems and concerns. At the same time, the media misses out on the significant emotional and relational bonding experience involved in sex. Married sex is so much richer than most of the media portrays.
>
> —*Kim, reflecting on sex with her husband*

❑ Completely safe because—

❑ Somewhat safe because—

❑ Completely unsafe because—

• What is it about your group that makes it fit that spot on the scale?

write here

SEXUAL IDENTITY

2

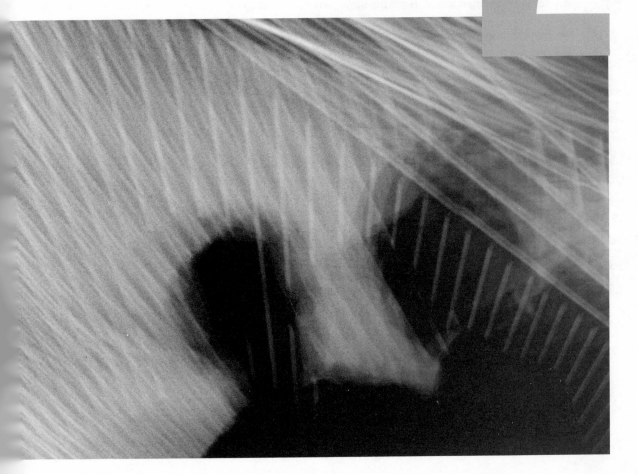

The first pages of the first book of the Bible say God made humans male and female. Women and men are a matched set—both are necessary for reproduction. Each benefits from the uniqueness of the other (we're speaking in general here—your mileage may vary depending on the quality of men and women you know). Anyway, that's sex, that's gender. Two X chromosomes deliver a female, an X and a Y produce a male. Different body chemistry, different physical structures—it's not rocket science.

Sexual identity is a different matter, though. Sexual identity is how we experience our sexuality, and what we think and how we feel about that. And then what we do about it. This has a lot to do with hormones—testosterone in boys and progesterone in girls. But it also has something to do with how we're treated by our families, friends, schools, mass media—the whole culture. That's what this chapter is mainly about.

From the day we're born, our families and friends and communities influence how we think about our sexuality. Women and men tell boys and girls how to act. We watch and learn from adults how it's really done. And we read, listen to the radio, go to the park, and watch television and movies. Bit by bit, we come to understand ourselves as males and females, which determines, for the most part, how we play and dress and talk and relate to other people.

And all is well in the neighborhood—until puberty hits like a flash flood and we're up to our hips in hormones.

Chubby boys grow angular. Their voices crack and drop, muscles mass and occasionally cramp in places where there didn't even used to be *places*, hair sprouts like patches of grass, unanticipated erections ambush them by day and erotic dreams produce involuntary ejaculations by night. It is, without question, a crazy time of life.

Skinny girls find their straight lines replaced by curving hips and bellies, their breasts bud and grow (evenly, they hope), they experience unexpected attention from older men, new hair grows on them too—though generally not as densely as on their brothers—and they cross their fingers, hoping against the odds they'll be safe at home when they menstruate the first time. These are exceedingly strange days for girls morphing into women.

Such explosive change blows sexual perceptions all over the map. Some of us don't seem too self-conscious about our sexuality. Others are conspicuously self-aware.

In the locker room, one boy saunters to the shower wearing nothing but a smile and a towel around his neck. The boy at the next locker wraps his towel around his waist like a kilt and holds on tight because there's a towel snatcher roaming the aisles of metal lockers. On the way, he passes a kid who doesn't need a towel because there's no way he's going near the shower.

In the classroom, a girl dressed for comfort is oblivious to the boy who sits behind her, transfixed by the curve of her bare shoulder. The girl in front of that girl is dressed to get attention and seems fully aware of her effect on boys—"She ain't got much," another girl whispers to her friend, "but it's all out there where they can get a look at it." At the back of the room, for reasons that are private and painful, another girl wears baggy clothes to hide her body.

And so it goes in adolescence; the unconscious and the hyperconscious, questioning, defining, and redefining our sexual identity.

What do you want to know about your sexual identity?

Here's a short list of things kids everywhere seem to wonder:

- Are my sexual responses normal?
- Why do I get nervous around people of the other gender?
- Why do I get turned on so easily?
- Do I get turned on like other people?
- Why do I feel guilty about my sexuality?
- Am I a sex fiend?
- Am I gay?
- Could I turn gay?

This list hasn't changed much in the last 50 years. Curiosity about homosexuality may have escalated a bit, but other than that, the list looks about the same.

Grown-up responses to these questions haven't changed much either. Christian adults who sit down for reasonable, biblically informed conversations about sexuality are few and far between. Half the church gets laryngitis when kids ask about these things. The other half talks louder.

Some adults are just plain uncomfortable talking about sexuality. So they answer a question with a question:

"Whadaya mean, 'Do you get turned on like other people?' You're not supposed to get turned on at all!"

"Why in the world would you even ask if you could turn into—one of those?"

One of the dirty little secrets about the church is that Christians don't always agree about sexuality. In fact, Christians can be downright disagreeable on the subject.

Take gender roles, for instance.

Some Christians believe being male means one thing and one thing only. And being female means the exact opposite. There are male jobs (thinking, heavy lifting, bringing home the bacon) and female jobs (cleaning, bearing and raising children, cooking the bacon) because—so the theory goes—that's the way God likes it. And anybody who crosses the behavioral divide has some explaining to do.

Other Christians believe the only differences between men and women are cultural and therefore nonbiblical, if not frankly *unbiblical*. They believe we invent what it means to act like women and men as we go along, from one culture to another. As far as these folks are concerned, people's gender is defined by their plumbing and wiring—but their behavior isn't (men can nurture without being feminine, and women can think without being masculine).

People in each of these two camps have been known to wonder if people in the other camp are even Christians. Jam all those opinions in one room and things get pretty noisy. Or very quiet. For a lot of Christians, it's easier to not have the conversation at all.

That's a mistake. Maybe this goes without saying, but if we don't decide what we think about sexual identity, someone else will tell us what to think. In fact, someone else is—loud and late into the night.

So we'd better.

like father, like son

WRITE ABOUT IT

Q: What are the most helpful messages about sexual identity you've received from your family?
  - What are the least helpful messages about sexual identity you've received from your family?

Q: What questions about sex could you talk about with your parents, siblings, or other family members you respect?

that's
gotta hurt

Sometimes tragic circumstances affect a person's sense of sexual identity.

THINK ABOUT IT

Q: What effect do you think physical disability might have on a person's sexual identity?

Q: What effect do you think verbal, emotional, or physical abuse might have on a person's sexual identity?
Talk about it.

Q: What effect do you think molestation or rape might have on a person's sexual identity? Talk about it.

Q: What effect do you think incest might have on a person's sexual identity?

Q: Are there other tragedies that might affect a person's sexual identity? Talk about it.

Q: Do you have any close friends or family who have suffered in any of these ways? How do you think they cope with the effects?
- What do you think they need?
- Do you think you would know how to help?

WRITE ABOUT IT

Q: To what degree would you say your sexual identity has been influenced by the following?

FACTOR	ZERO	SOME	TONS
PHYSICAL DISABILITY			
VERBAL, EMOTIONAL, OR PHYSICAL ABUSE			
SEXUAL MOLESTATION OR RAPE			
INCEST			
YOU NAME IT:_____			

Q: Apart from physical challenges, if you've been the victim of any abuse, who knows about that besides you and the person or persons responsible?
  • If nobody else knows, what do you have to gain or lose by keeping it to yourself?

Q: Whether or not you've told another human, there is someone who already knows: God. What do you think he might have to say to you about what you've been through and how that's affecting you now? If you're not sure, ask a Christian adult—like a parent, teacher, or youth pastor—who might be able to help you figure it out.

God: the before and the after

GOD'S-EYE VIEW

Here's some background on Genesis 1:25-2:1.
    This is the beginning of the story of sexual identity. In fact it's the beginning of the story of everything human. Read through the passage carefully. You may be surprised about how much bad stuff happened as a result of human rebellion against God.

THINK ABOUT IT

Look at Genesis 1:25-2:1.

Q: What do you think are the big ideas in this passage? Why do those seem important to you?

Q: Can you see any difference in the design criteria for animals in verse 25 and humans in verses 26 and 27? If so, what is it?

Q: What do you think about verse 27?
  • What do you think that means? Why?

WRITE ABOUT IT

Q: Can you identify any glimpses of God's image in you? What are they?
  • How do you believe that image is affected by your own sin and wrongdoing?

GOD'S-EYE VIEW

Some folks believe sin has completely obliterated the image of God in humans. Others believe it's only hidden it, as a blanket can hide something special or valuable. Either way, sin has created a problem for us—a problem so big that only God can help us.

> God created man in his own image, in the image of God he created him; male and female he created them.

> The most common word used for *sin* in the Bible means *missing the mark*. Imagine you're holding a bow and arrow, ready to shoot at a target. Your aim is off and your shot veers right or left of the target. Well, in this case, the target is God's will for us, which is to love and serve him first and others second. And boy howdy, do we miss that target a lot.

Read 2 Corinthians 5:17.

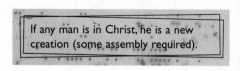
If any man is in Christ, he is a new creation (some assembly required).

Q: Okay, but wait a minute. If you're a new creation, why do you still struggle with sin issues (sexual stuff in particular)?

Q: How is it possible that the reality of you being a brand new creation in Christ coexists with the ever-present reality that you are sinful, broken, and struggling?

Q: Paul seems to address this very tension in Romans 7:14-28. He seems fully aware of the inner struggle between doing what is right and what is wrong, and yet points to a rescuer in Romans 7:24. Who is that rescuer?

Q: It's true that Jesus rescues us from sin when we ask him to take over our lives and be our Savior and Lord. But how do you need him to rescue you from your sin and sexual struggles even *after* you've committed your life to him?

mercy + judgment

THINK ABOUT IT

Look at Romans 1:15-2:15.

Q: What stands out for you in this passage?

Q: According to this passage, what are some things that happen when people resist God?

Q: What would you say has changed since these words were written?

For what it's worth, when verse 32 uses the phrase "those who do such things deserve death," the original language means those who do such things *repeatedly and habitually* deserve death.

Q: Do you believe that's significant? Why or why not?

Q: What do you think Romans 2:4 means?

GOD'S-EYE VIEW

A thought about Romans 1:15-2:15.

When we do the wrong things, our sexuality is devastated along with the rest of us—soul, mind, spirit and relationships. God can and will redeem it all, renewing us in the bright morning of our youth or rescuing us at death's gate, by the skin of our teeth. Because of God's mercy and kindness, you and I have no excuse for waiting one more heartbeat to surrender our will and our life to the Creator. And neither does anyone else.

Q: Do you see things in this passage that describe events in your life? Who else knows about this? Is there someone who should know? Why?
  • Do you see anything in this passage that's repeated and habitual for you? Do you believe you're in any danger? Why?

teenage
~~Jesus~~

THINK ABOUT IT

Q: Read Luke 2:52. What do you think is the significance of the statement that *Jesus grew*?
  • Do you think the way Jesus grew is a better model for boys or for girls?

WRITE ABOUT IT

Q: What signs of personal growth do you see in the last year?

  • in wisdom—

  • in stature—

  • in favor with God—

  • in favor with man—

Q: In what ways do you think you need to grow in the months ahead?

  • in wisdom—

  • in stature—

  • in favor with God—

  • in favor with man—

Q: Are there obstacles to your growth in any of these areas? What are they?

Q: Do you know someone who might be able to help you in one of these areas? Why?

fruit: a manly meal
or a feminine delight?

Q: Do you think most people seem confused about what's masculine and what's feminine? Explain your answer.
  • Do you ever feel confused about what's masculine and what's feminine?

Q: Do you think of the attributes in Galatians 5:22-23 as more masculine or more feminine or more human?

FRUIT OF THE SPIRIT	MORE MASCULINE BECAUSE—	MORE FEMININE BECAUSE—	MORE HUMAN BECAUSE—
LOVE			
JOY			
PEACE			
PATIENCE			
KINDNESS			
GOODNESS			
FAITHFULNESS			
GENTLENESS			
SELF-CONTROL			

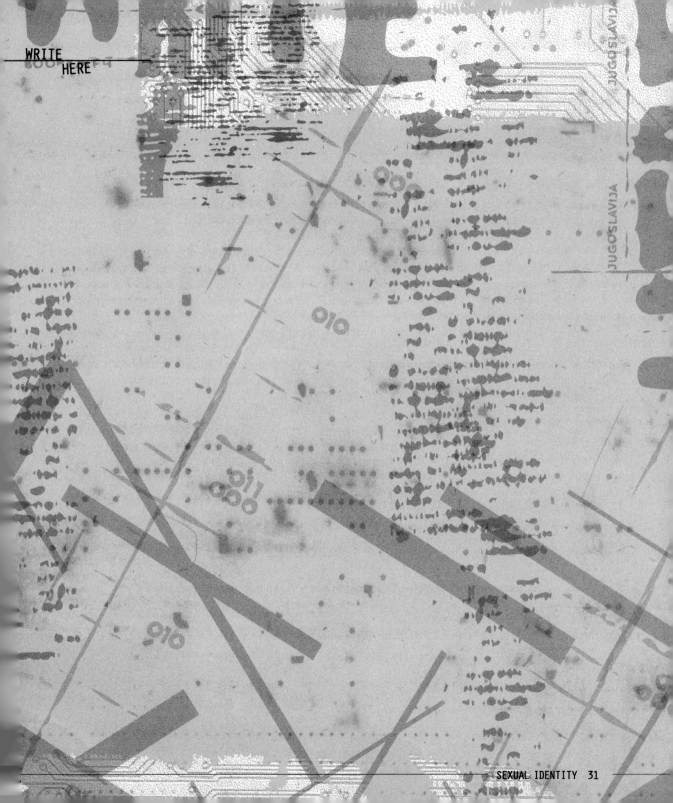

Q: Think back on the past year. Which of the fruit of the Spirit would you say are more obvious in your life today than a year ago? How do you feel about that?
- Do you think any of the Spirit's fruit is less obvious in your life than a year ago? Explain your answer.

GOD'S-EYE VIEW

A thought about Galatians 5:22-23—

Jesus combined what we call masculine and feminine traits in a comfortable balance of humanness. He hugged children and spoke up for them (Mark 10:13-16), he got physical with merchants who exploited poor people in the temple (John 2:13-22), he was tough on people who were full of themselves (John 5:41-47), he cried over the grief of a friend (John 11:35). Jesus was not a stereotypical, testosterone-crazed man, and he wasn't a sissy. In a culture where children were disposable and women would have been second-class citizens if they'd been allowed to be citizens at all, Jesus respected children and treated women as equals.

And the spirit of Jesus, the Holy Spirit, produces fruit in every believer's life—because with the fruit of the Spirit, gender has nothing to do with anything. The fruit of the Spirit is love, joy, peace, patience, kindness, goodness, faithfulness, gentleness, self-control—legal in all 50 states and Puerto Rico. God's Spirit nullifies "boys will be boys" and "women—can't live with 'em, can't live without 'em." The Holy Spirit replaces roughness with gentleness and transforms compulsiveness into self-control.

In our culture women may be considered masculine and men may be thought feminine for exhibiting characteristics that are merely godly. It breaks my heart—on those days when it doesn't make me angry—that these characterizations are about as common inside the family of God as outside. We can't control what outsiders say about us, but shame on us for choosing cultural stereotypes over the whole basket of the fruit of the Spirit. That's just plain wrong.

WRITE ABOUT IT

Q: Do you ever wonder if you're as masculine (or feminine) as you're supposed to be?

Q: Who are the best models of masculinity you know?
- What makes their masculinity appealing?

Q: Who are the best models of femininity you know?
- What makes their femininity appealing?

Q: What do you think the best models of masculinity and femininity have in common with each other?
- How are they different?

Q: With whom can you talk about masculinity, femininity, and the evidence of the Spirit's presence in your life?

WRITE HERE

WRITE HERE

the "h" word

Q: Which statement best describes your opinion?

❑ I believe homosexuals are born, not made—it runs in the family genes.

❑ I believe homosexuals are made by their environments, not born.

❑ I believe homosexuals are homosexual for many reasons, not just one.

❑ I believe homosexuals have perverted thinking.

❑ I believe homosexuality is a birth defect, like spina bifida or cystic fibrosis.

❑ I don't know why some people are homosexual.

❑ The reason I believe some people are homosexuals is—

Okay, now add a *because* to your answer.

❑ I agreed that homosexuals are born, not made, because—

❑ I agreed that homosexuals are made, not born, because—

❑ I agreed that I don't know why some people are homosexual because—

Q: Where do you think you got your ideas about homosexual identity?

> At the time of this writing, the research regarding the influence of biological forces in the development of sexual identity (especially homosexual identity) is inconclusive.

THINK ABOUT IT

Q: Why do you think homosexuality is such a volatile issue in our culture?

Q: Are you well acquainted with someone who describes herself as a homosexual?

Q: Homosexual relationships seem increasingly acceptable in our society. Do you agree that in our society (and maybe even among some of your friends), it's kinda cool these days to be gay? If you agree, why do you think it's this way?

Q: What do you think Scripture says about this issue? Do you know any passages offhand that relate to homosexuality?

GOD'S-EYE VIEW

If you need some hints on biblical passages, try Genesis 19:1-17, Leviticus 18:1-30, Romans 1:18-2:15, and 1 Corinthians 6:9-11.

Q: How do these Scripture verses color your view of homosexuality?

Q: It's been said that given the other sins described in many of these passages, homosexuality is no worse than any other sin, including heterosexual lust. What do you think of that argument?

Q: Do you think there's a difference between homosexual curiosity and homosexual identity? Talk about that.
- How about between homosexual tendencies and acting on those tendencies?

Q: Some churches have the reputation for being unwelcoming to homosexuals, insisting that they change their lifestyles before they become a part of the community. Other churches welcome homosexuals just as they are and don't require that they change their behavior or lifestyle at all. Still others welcome homosexuals into the church community but exclude them from leadership. What do you think of these three positions?
- What do you think God thinks of them?

> It's taken a long time to realize that God is not the enemy of my enemies—he's not the enemy of his enemies.
> —Martin Niemuller, German pastor imprisoned by Nazis

Q: Some Christians believe that ministry to homosexuals begins with loving them and getting to know them. Others believe it begins with telling them they're disobeying God. What do you think of these two starting points?
- If you had a friend who was homosexual (and many of you do), how would you want to start ministering to them?

write here

WRITE HERE

WRITE HERE

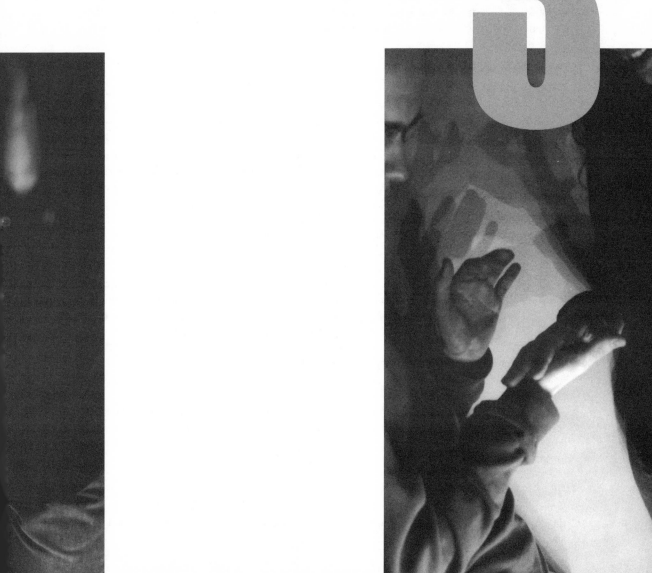

INTIMACY

3

INTIMACY

Intimacy grows between people who trust each other with their deepest natures. Intimacy rejects fakery and shortcuts. There's no such thing as instant intimacy. Instant attraction, yes. Instant crushes, of course. But real intimacy takes time. You can tell you're in an intimate relationship if you both choose being real instead of faking it, being warm instead of cool, understanding instead of judging.

But intimacy is not a feeling, it's a condition. Intimacy takes time and attention and energy. To some people, that sounds a lot like work. So sometimes they do things to *feel* intimate even if they really aren't. It's rumored that some girls have sex to feel intimate. It's also rumored that some boys fake intimacy in order to get sex.

It doesn't take a genius to understand what happens when people pretend to be intimate—you get Intimacy Lite. Less filling, but still intoxicating in sufficient quantities.

It also doesn't take a genius to understand why people might settle for Intimacy Lite. True intimacy is risky. Being intimate means facing the possibility of rejection and embarrassment. If I reveal the truth about me, I risk the possibility that you'll say, "Eww, that's creepy." Which, needless to say, is painful.

That's why intimacy is so hard—it's a high-risk investment. And every successful investor knows that Rule One is *Don't risk more than you can afford to lose*. So, after we get hurt a couple of times, most of us learn to lie back and play it safe, investing a little of our true selves but not enough to risk a serious loss. It's a good strategy. Except for the fact that humans need intimacy whether we want it or not.

Right from the start (Genesis 2:18), God declared that humans ought not to be alone—we need help to make it. God says, plain as day, it's not good for humans to be isolated. Most of us know instinctively that God is right about this. Risky as it is, what people crave perhaps more than anything else is authentic intimacy.

But turns out that sex is a handy substitute for authentic intimacy.

There's no question that sex feels intimate. Breathing the same air, sharing the same space, being glued together sexually—*glued together* is how the Bible puts it when two people are united as "one flesh" (Genesis 2:24; Matthew 19:5-6; Mark 10:7-8; 1 Corinthians 6:16; Ephesians 5:31—the words translated *cleave* in the King James and *united* in the NIV, mean *to glue together*). It's hard to get any closer than that.

But when a sexual relationship comes unglued, so do the feelings.

PHASE 1—GUESS WHO

The mess begins when someone—let's call her Sophie—tries to figure out what sort of person the sort of person she wants to go out with wants to go out with. (Are you following this?)

Generally, Sophie has someone in mind—Joaquin or Billy Joe or Shaquille or Haig, could be anyone—because he's cute or looks like he needs rescuing or whatever.

PHASE 2—MASQUERADE

Sophie figures out what Haig wants and says, "I can be that." Then she fakes her way to romance. Sooner or later, directly or indirectly, Sophie tells a lie to maintain the masquerade. It's doomed from the start; anyone can see that.

PHASE 3—GETTING SERIOUS

This is easy to spot. Just look for two high school juniors acting like married people, except they live with their parents. Neither can make plans without consulting the other, they cross the borders of married sexual behavior, they can't talk about where they'd like to be in five years without somebody getting hurt feelings, they buy stuff together. Sophie finds it's easier to "make love"—which makes her feel close, temporarily at least, to Haig—than to talk seriously with him, which is frustrating in the extreme.

PHASE 4—THE CINDERELLA SYNDROME

Eventually, the clock strikes 12, and Sophie turns into the poor stepsister. It's humiliating and sad and she feels she's lost something she can't replace. She's distracted (or intensely focused), she can't sleep (or can't wake up), she gains weight (or loses weight). For a while, Sophie wonders if she'll make it. But, after a few weeks, she thinks it's probably just as well because she never really enjoyed pretending to be a Cow-Punk-Choir-Girl-Skate-Rat anyway. Haig was a jerk—how could she not see that? Sophie makes a mental note not to get so emotionally involved next time. If there is a next time.

Then one day, out of the blue, Sophie wonders—again—what sort of person the sort of person she wants to go out with wants to go out with. (You following this?)

No wonder some people try to drain the emotion from sexuality.

But it doesn't work. No matter what people say about casual sex, in the end, it's quite personal. If you don't believe it, keep watching.

Now here's a funny thing. For a culture that wants to take the intimacy out of sex, we're awfully busy sexualizing intimacy these days. Many in our culture believe intimacy inevitably leads to sex. "You can't get that close to people without going farther," they say—and by *going farther* they mean sexually. This is intimacy as foreplay, and it's highly toxic to otherwise healthy friendships. (Have you noticed how many people get sexually involved with their close friends—and how they tend to drift apart afterward?) There goes the possibility of friendship between men and women. Too bad. The Bible

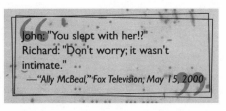

John: "You slept with her!?"
Richard: "Don't worry; it wasn't intimate."
—"Ally McBeal," Fox Television, May 15, 2000

describes us—Christians, at least—as brothers and sisters. Sorry, but there are things healthy brothers and sisters don't do.

Even same-gender intimacy is threatened by the assumption—or fear—that people can't get close without getting busy. Not everybody makes that assumption, not by a long shot. It's crazy and unfair. But it's there like a rumor, isolating people, making them uncomfortable and suspicious and separate. Again—too bad.

It's not supposed to be like this. Because it's no good for people to be isolated. God said so.

intimacy

THINK ABOUT IT

Q: Where do you think most people get their ideas about intimacy?
 • What do you think most people mean when they use the term intimacy?

WRITE ABOUT IT

Q: What's your definition of intimacy?
 • How did you come up with that definition?

Q: Do you think sex equals intimacy?

❏ Absolutely not because— ❏ Maybe, maybe not because— ❏ Absolutely because—

best buds

Here's some background on 1 Samuel 20:1-42.

David has been anointed king of Israel by Samuel, though officially Saul is still in power. Saul seems to have a love-hate relationship with David—approving of his conquests in battle, yet jealous of his successes. Whatever Saul does to harm David becomes David's advantage. Saul keeps trying to kill David by throwing spears at him (1 Samuel 18 and 19), and David's success at evading him only increases Saul's anxiety. Saul gives his daughter Michal to David as a wife, hoping she'll trap him. But instead Michal falls in love with David and helps him escape from Saul's murderous trap.

Now read the plan David and Jonathan (Saul's son and David's best friend) make together.

THINK ABOUT IT

Look at 1 Samuel 20:1-42.

Q: If someone handed you 1 Samuel 20 and asked you to circle the verses that show the intimacy between David and Jonathan, what verses would you circle?

Q: Do you believe friendship with someone of the same gender is essentially different than friendship with someone of the opposite gender?

Q: Do you believe it's okay to only have friends of the same gender only? Why?
  • Do you believe it's okay to only have friends of the opposite gender? Why?

Q: Do you believe it was okay for Jonathan to deceive his father under the circumstances described in 1 Samuel 20?
  • When, if ever, do you think friendship comes before family? Why?

GOD'S-EYE VIEW

Look at 1 Samuel 20:13-15.

Q: Jonathan's phrase, "May the Lord be with you as he had been with my father" reveals Jonathan's expectation that David has a special calling from God and will have quite a dynasty, probably even as the king. But, since Jonathan is Saul's son, he is supposed to be the next king. What does Jonathan's willingness to surrender his right to be king say about his friendship with David?
  • Do you think many people share that kind of intimacy? Why?
  • What would that kind of friendship be worth to you?

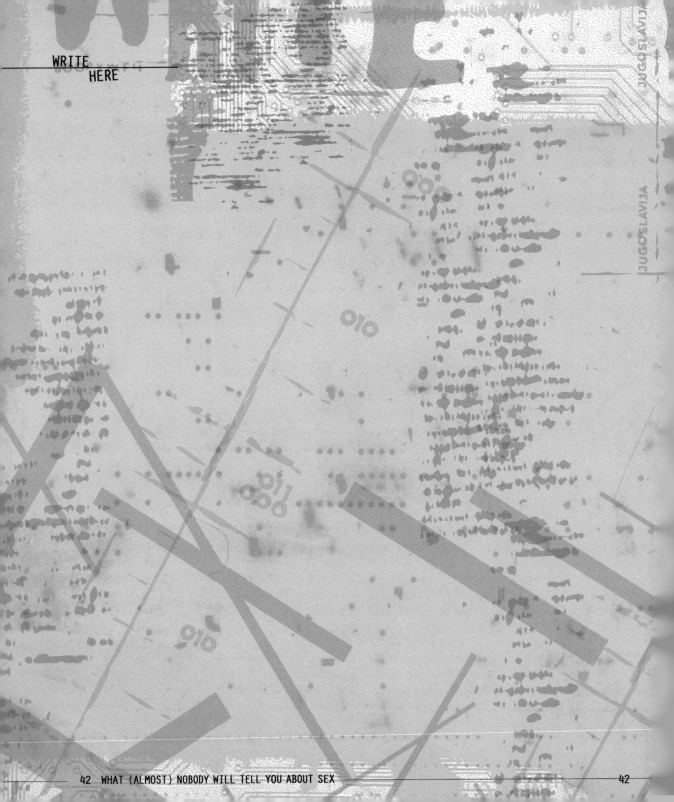

Q: Who are your closest friends?
  • What makes them so close?

Look at I Corinthians 13:4-7.

Q: Compare I Samuel 20 with these verses in I Corinthians 13. How do you think Jonathan and David stack up in the comparison?
  • Compare your closest friendships with I Corinthians 13:4-7. How do you think you stack up?

four loves

Greek, the language in which The New Testament was written, has several different words for *love*. Two of them appear prominently in the New Testament.

  • *Agape* (uh-GAW-pay) is the unconditional love God shows us and the unconditional love we can likewise show others (see Mark 12:31).
  • *Philia* (fill-EE-uh) is affectionate love for a friend (see Romans 12:10), from which we get the name *Philadelphia*.
  • *Eros* (AIR-oss) is sexual love, from which we get the word *erotic*. The word *eros* doesn't appear in the New Testament, but the idea is all over the Song of Songs.
  • *Storge* (STORE-gay) is the love shared in healthy families. This word is also absent in the New Testament but present in spirit.

Q: How would you describe the love you show your family right now?

Q: How would you describe the love you show your friends right now?

Q: How would you describe the unconditional love you show others right now?

Q: How would you describe your erotic love right now?

Q: Which of the four loves is closest to where you think it should be right now?

Q: Which kind of love needs the most work in your life?

> [Love] is called Agape in the New Testament to distinguish it from Eros (sexual love), Storge (family affection), and Philia (friendship). So there are four kinds of love, all good in their proper place, but Agape is the best because it is the kind God has for us and is good in all circumstances.
> —C. S. Lewis, Letters of C.S. Lewis
> (Harcourt Brace Jovanovich)

GOD'S-EYE VIEW

Okay, maybe you're thinking unconditional love is hard to show. You're right. Only God can show it all the time. However, as we experience his unconditional love more and more, it becomes easier to show it to others.

Q: Do you think a relationship can experience different kinds of loves at different times? Explain your answer.

Q: Have you seen or experienced a shift from friendly love to erotic love? If so, what happened?
- Have you seen or experienced a shift from erotic love to friendly love? What happened?
- What good and bad things happen in a friendship when *eros* love is expressed?

WRITE ABOUT IT

Q: If someone asked you how to keep a healthy balance of the four loves in a friendship, what would you tell that person?
- If someone asked the same question about a dating relationship, what would you tell that person?

one anothering

WRITE ABOUT IT

Circle the one another commands from these passages in the Bible. There are a lot more than these, but we ran out of room. You can add to the list

Do not steal. Do not lie. Do not deceive one another (Leviticus 19:11).

Salt is good, but if it lose its saltiness, how can you make it salty again? Have salt in yourselves, and be at peace with each other (Mark 9:50).

A new command I give you: Love one another. As I have loved you, so you must love one another (John 13:34).

Accept one another, then, just as Christ accepted you, in order to bring praise to God (Romans 15:7).

You, my brothers, were called to be free. But do not use your freedom to indulge the sinful nature; rather, serve one another in love (Galatians 5:13).

Be completely humble and gentle; be patient, bearing with one another in love (Ephesians 4:2).

Be kind and compassionate to one another, forgiving each other, just as in Christ God forgave you (Ephesians 4:32).

And let us consider how we may spur one another on toward love and good deeds (Hebrews 10:24).

Therefore confess your sins to each other and pray for each other so that you may be healed (James 5:16).

WRITE HERE

WRITE HERE

WRITE HERE

THINK ABOUT IT

Q: What do you think is the point in all this one-anothering?

Q: Which one-another commands do you think could realistically happen in a friendship?
- Which of the one-another commands do you think could realistically happen in a dating relationship? Why?
- What could get in the way of that kind of commitment?
- Where do you think it's easier for people to one-another—in a friendship or a dating relationship? Explain your answer.
- If someone could one-another you back in a dating relationship or a friendship, what kinds of spiritual qualities would that person have?

WRITE ABOUT IT

Q: Review the one-anothering list and circle some things you'd like to try this week.
- Next to any command you circled, write someone's name and an idea of how you could act on it.
- What do you need from God to carry out your plan?

The yoke's on you

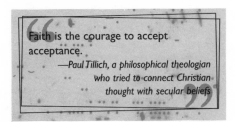

" Faith is the courage to accept acceptance.
—Paul Tillich, a philosophical theologian who tried to connect Christian thought with secular beliefs "

THINK ABOUT IT

Look at 2 Corinthians 6:14-18.

Q: What stands out to you in these verses? Why do you think that's significant?

GOD'S-EYE VIEW

When Paul uses the image of yoking together in 2 Corinthians, it refers to two farm animals in a double harness that are so incompatible they can't possibly pull together (see Deuteronomy 22:10). The name *Belial*, in verse 15, comes from Jewish literature. *Belial* refers to a personalized force opposed to God.

Q: Have you ever seen a Christian in an incompatible yoke? You might even be thinking of yourself here.
- What happened between them in the long run?
- What did you learn from that? How does it relate to Paul's words?

WRITE ABOUT IT

Q: What arguments have you heard regarding why it's not okay for believers and unbelievers to date?

Q: What arguments have you heard regarding why it's okay for believers and unbelievers to date?

Q: Bottom line—how do you feel about believers and unbelievers dating each other? Why?

Look at 1 Corinthians 9:19-23.

One possibility is that Paul is talking about two different kinds of relationships in these passages. In 1 Corinthians 9 Paul is talking about his work as an apostle. In 2 Corinthians 6 he seems to be talking about essential lifestyle links between believers and nonbelievers—especially the kinds that can pull you away from God, just the way it was happening in the city of Corinth.

Q: The image of our bodies as temples of the Holy Spirit is fairly common among Christians. What does Paul seem to believe it means in this passage?

Q: How does having our body as God's temple relate to being unequally yoked?

Q: Have you reached any conclusions about unequal yoking? If so, what are they?

to wed or not to wed

GOD'S-EYE VIEW

A bit of background on 1 Corinthians 7:25-40—
   When Paul wrote 1 Corinthians, he was trying to help the new church in Corinth handle the problems it was facing. There is some specific crisis in Corinth (see 7:26), so keep in mind that his recommendations might not apply to all times and all situations.

THINK ABOUT IT

Q: According to this passage, how do married people live differently from single people?
   • Is being single better than being married? Why or why not?

Q: Are there advantages or disadvantages to being married that Paul doesn't mention?

Q: How many advantages to singleness do you find in this passage? If so, what are they?
   • Do you think there are disadvantages to singleness that Paul doesn't describe? What are they?

Q: Do you think it's possible to be married and still serve God wholeheartedly? Why?

Q: Do you think it's possible to be single for the rest of your life and still feel good about yourself? Given how Paul talks about singleness, why do you think we even have to ask the question today?

Q: How has your relationship with God been different when you were dating someone as opposed to when you weren't?

Q: If you could plan out your life, at what age would you want to transition from being single to married—if at all?
- Have you seriously considered remaining single for your whole life?

Q: How do messages from others affect your attitudes about remaining single?

Q: Do you have any sense about what God may have in mind for you as a married person or a single person? If so, write as many specific things as you can.

they kissed dating goodbye

Some people believe there's no room for erotic expression of any kind before people are married. In other words they believe you shouldn't date in the contemporary sense before you are committed to marry. In this scenario you'd remain friends with someone, getting to know them better and better, but not dating them or getting physically involved.

> Language has created the word "loneliness" to express the pain of being alone, and the word "solitude" to express the glory of being alone.
> —Paul Tillich, a philosophical theologian who tried to connect Christian thought with secular beliefs

WRITE ABOUT IT

Q: Take five minutes to write as many reasons as you can why you believe that's a genuinely brilliant idea.
- Now, take five minutes to write as many reasons as you can why that's a genuinely dumb idea.

THINK ABOUT IT

Q: Suppose you kissed dating goodbye. Would that create problems for you?
- Would it solve any problems if you kissed dating goodbye?

Q: Suppose you choose to date in a more or less normal pattern from now on. Would that create problems for you?
- Would dating like everybody else solve any problems for you?

WRITE ABOUT IT

Q: How compatible do you think Christianity is with American-style dating?

Q: Do you think men and women can really be friends? Why or why not?
- What does dating do for you that an intimate friendship doesn't—positively and negatively?

Q: Is there anyone in your life who knows how you feel about dating?
- If not, who could you trust to tell the truth about dating?
- What do you have to gain or lose by telling the truth about this? Why?

breaking up (is so very hard to do)

THINK ABOUT IT

Q: Think about the messiest breakup you've ever seen.
- Why do you believe things went so badly?
- What did you learn from that breakup?

Q: What seem to be the most common ingredients in breakups that go poorly?
- Do you believe those problems could be prevented? How?

WRITE ABOUT IT

Q: Describe the nicest, cleanest, most godly breakup you've seen.
- What factors do you believe made that less messy than other breakups?
- What did you learn from that breakup?

Q: In general, what do you believe it takes for a breakup to go well?
- What do you believe is the biggest barrier to that?

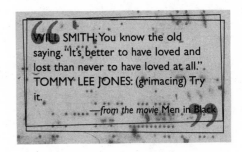

> WILL SMITH: You know the old saying. "It's better to have loved and lost than never to have loved at all." TOMMY LEE JONES: (grimacing) Try it.
> —from the movie Men in Black

Q: Let's say the greatest emotional pain you ever endured was a 10. Now circle the number that describes the most recent breakup you've had.

1 —— 2 —— 3 —— 4 —— 5 —— 6 —— 7 —— 8 —— 9 —— 10

- How long did it take you to get over that pain? (Or how do long do you think it will take?)
- Where do you think God was in all that?

Q: How do you think having sex affects the breakup? Does it make it harder? Easier? The same?

love stories

Spend some time with a parent, an uncle, an aunt, or a grandparent you admire and trust. Ask these questions (videotape them or make an audio tape if you want to save their responses outside your brain)—

- How did your love story begin?
- What did you share in common at the beginning?
- What did you come to love about the other person?
- What did your love bring you that you didn't already have?
- What has it cost you to love?
- How did the two of you decide to marry?
- What changed when you got married?
- What do you value about your spouse now that you didn't before?

WRITE ABOUT IT

Now back to you—

Q: What do you respect about those people's love relationships? Why?

Q: What do you believe you would have to do to get what they have?
- Is there anything that could keep you from getting that? Why?

Q: If you talked with someone other than your parents, how do you think these love stories compare to your parents' relationship? How do you feel about that?
- If you marry, how do you think your relationship with your spouse will be different than your parents' relationship? Why?

Q: As you think about your future, are there any fresh commitments you need to make about your life? If so, what are they?

I'd been dating a guy—we'll call him Brian—for about two months. His mom asked me to help her plan a surprise birthday party for him. By the time the party ended, it was really late—too late for his mom to drive me home—so she asked me if I just wanted to spend the night in their guest room. I called my mom and explained that I'd have my own room and everything, so both she and I thought it would be okay.

About 20 minutes after I turned the lights off, I heard the door open. It was Brian. He came and lay down next to me on the bed. He explained that he loved me and that he wanted to make love to me. To be honest, even though I had grown up in church, I wanted it too.

That night we had sex. I went home the next morning feeling a little bit happy but mostly really dirty.

He broke up with me three days later.

—Jenna, a 15-year-old

---

write here

WRITE HERE

WRITE HERE

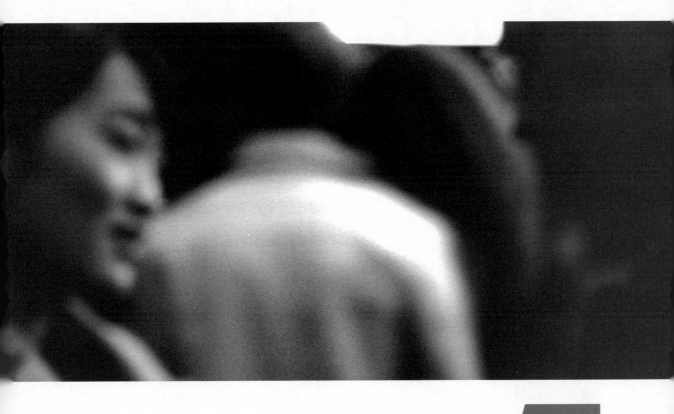

DESIRE

4

Desire is good. Except when it's bad.

Think about it. Desire drives one person to sacrifice herself in pursuit of a cure for AIDS. Desire drives another person to indulge in behavior that spreads HIV.

Desire is tricky that way.

Healthy desire generates commitment and propels accomplishment. Unhealthy desire, on the other hand (and there's always that other hand), fuels lust. And lust, as the book of James says, gives birth to sin—which, when it's full-grown, gives birth to death (James 1:15). Yikes!

Learning to cultivate healthy desires and avoid being seduced by unhealthy desires is what this chapter is about.

And it's not hard to see what unhealthy desire does to relationships. Let's face it—most of us are young and inexperienced, no matter how mature or sophisticated we appear to be. Look for these telltale signs in others.

> I've never really been mad at God—
> God just has the job I want.

- They get selfish and pushy when the one thing they desire is the very thing (or experience or relationship) they can't have. Watch for aggressive or obnoxious behavior (not hostile, necessarily, but still disagreeable).

- Those who feel they're entitled to more start to take more. Watch for foot-dragging, lateness, incomplete follow-through, testing limits, whining, and other passive resistance. Listen for reports from their friends of loyalty tests, tongue-lashings, and ultimatums.

- When people think something is being withheld from them, they can get sneaky and secretive. Look for lying, cover-ups, and burning bridges.

And look for someone on the other side of the relationship who says (sooner than later, we hope), "Who needs that? I'm outta here."

This is a critical moment. The young man or woman with the courage to withdraw from someone whose desire is out of control needs support and encouragement. That person's commitment to health will almost certainly be tested.

The one struggling with unhealthy desire also needs care. Because the next stop may be isolation, followed by obsession, then perversion. If that person is male, he is more likely to take his own life at this time than at any other time during adolescence. So try not to leave him high and dry.

In any event, look for signs of withdrawal, isolation, substance abuse, violence, and other high-risk behavior. Use your network of friends to draw that person out. Give him an invitation to vent feelings *without* giving false hopes of rekindling the flame (remember, he was playing with fire to begin with). If you detect signs of obsession—telephone hang-ups, stalking, self-mutilation—consider bringing in a trustworthy adult (not someone who'll freak, someone who'll help).

The apostle Paul told his flock in Corinth that God used some kind of persistent problem (he didn't give details) to keep him from getting conceited. Paul says he pleaded with God to take it away again and again, but God said, "My grace is sufficient for you, for my power is made perfect in weakness" (2 Corinthians 12:9). So, Paul said, he came to delight in weakness. He's in a fairly small club—because of his delight, not his weakness.

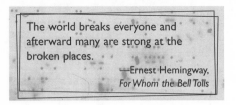

The world breaks everyone and afterward many are strong at the broken places.
—Ernest Hemingway,
For Whom the Bell Tolls

Some Bible teachers say Paul was referring to some kind of physical weakness, like progressive blindness, and maybe that's right. But lay this passage next to Paul's lament in Romans 7 and see what you get.

> I know that nothing good lives in me, that is, in my sinful nature. For I have the desire to do what is good, but I cannot carry it out. For what I do is not the good I want to do; no, the evil I do not want to do—this I keep on doing. Now if I do what I do not want to do, it is no longer I who do it, but it is sin living in me that does it. So I find this law at work: When I want to do good, evil is right there with me. For in my inner being I delight in God's law; but I see another law at work in the members of my body, waging war against the law of my mind and making me a prisoner of the law of sin at work within my members. What a wretched man I am! Who will rescue me from this body of death? Thanks be to God—through Jesus Christ our Lord! So then, I myself in my mind am a slave to God's law, but in the sinful nature a slave to the law of sin.
>
> **—Romans 7:18-25**

Again, some teachers explain this away, saying he was talking about life before he was a Christian. But the evidence suggests another possibility. It's possible that Paul struggled with an unhealthy desire so powerful only Jesus could overcome it. If that's true, Paul wasn't alone in his struggle with desire, and the rest of us shouldn't be surprised when we struggle. Because desire is tricky that way.

guess who's sexually active

THINK ABOUT IT

Q: Many surveys indicate that a large percentage of teens are sexually active. In your experience and given your circle of friends, do you think that's the case?

GOD'S-EYE VIEW

From another point of view, there's no such thing as a sexually inactive person—because beginning with adolescence, everyone deals with his or her own bubbling hormones and more or less intense sexual desires. Everybody is sexually active in the sense that they're growing and making choices about what to do sexually.

Q: What do you think about that? Why?

WRITE HERE

WRITE HERE

WRITE HERE

WRITE HERE

Q: When do you remember first having sexual thoughts and desires?
  • How did that make you feel?

WRITE ABOUT IT

Q: In what ways are you sexually active?
  • How do you typically respond to your sexual desires?
  • How do you feel about your typical response?

desire versus need

THINK ABOUT IT

Q: Do you believe your sexual hunger is a *desire* or a *need*?
  • Where did you get your ideas about that? How reliable do you think that is?

Q: Do you think girls have stronger sexual desires than guys—or vice versa? What makes you think that?

WRITE ABOUT IT

Q: What do you think is the biggest challenge in controlling sexual choices?

Q: What kind of sexual desires are you experiencing these days?

Q: Who can you talk to about these desires?

Q: What do you think the Bible says about these desires, fears, or other urges? Why do you think that?

> In one survey of teenage boys and girls, 63 percent judged the male sex drive as "uncontrollable," while only 13 percent judged the female sex drive as "uncontrollable."
> —S. Moore and D. Rosenthal, *Sexuality in Adolescence (Routledge)*

> A common theme among teens is that their sexual desire is so strong they just can't stop themselves. Is it so strong that if their parents walked in on what they were doing, they still wouldn't be able to stop?

choices, choices everywhere

THINK ABOUT IT

Look at 2 Samuel 11:1-17.

Q: Can you identify points at which David might have made a different and better decision in this story?
  • What were David's options when he first saw Bathsheba? Why do you think he made that choice?
  • What were David's options when he found out Bathsheba was married? Why do you think he chose as he did?
  • What were David's options when he found out Bathsheba was pregnant and her husband was off fighting for his country? Why do you think he chose what he chose?

Look at David's own words in 1 Samuel 21:5.

Q: What were David's options when Bathsheba's husband refused to go home to her while his soldiers were still in the field? Why do you think David made the choice he made?

David eventually repented in 2 Samuel 12, but the damage had been done. Now look at James 1:13-15.

Q: Why do you think James used sexual imagery in his description of temptation?

Q: What is the outcome of the seduction and birth of sin?
  • What examples of that outcome do you see in the story of David? You might want to read 2 Samuel 12:1-23 before you answer.

Q: Why is it that even when people know the right thing to do, they sometimes choose to do the wrong thing— or is that just me?

GOD'S-EYE VIEW

Knowing what we should do, but then struggling to be able to do it. That's not a problem only you face—it's common to every follower of Christ. Even Paul faced it. You don't believe us? Look up Romans 7:7-25 and see for yourself. Pay special attention to Romans 7:24-25. Who's going to rescue Paul? There's only one who can do it— Jesus Christ.

WRITE ABOUT IT

Q: What sexual desires are you experiencing right now?

Q: What did you choose to do the last time you faced those desires? Why?
  • What do you want to choose next time you face those desires? How does Romans 7:24-25 help you know what to do?

hang on to your hormones

THINK ABOUT IT

Look at Genesis 39:1-23.

Q: What do you like best about this story? Why?

GOD'S-EYE VIEW

Joseph must have been pretty good looking because the Bible, which seldom refers to physical appearances, describes him in Genesis 39:6 as "well-built and handsome." It must have run in the family—the only other person

in the Old Testament praised for both her figure and face was Joseph's mom, Rachel, who is described in Genesis 29:17 as "lovely in form and beautiful."

Q: Put yourself in Joseph's place. You're a talented, good looking slave kid who'd no doubt like to hang onto your job—not to mention your head. What would you think and feel if your owner's wife came on to you?

GOD'S-EYE VIEW

In prison Joseph eventually met people who connected him with the pharaoh. Seeing how talented Joseph was—and it didn't hurt that God gave Joseph insight into his plans for Egypt—the pharaoh placed him in charge of the government, where Joseph prepared the whole nation to survive a drought that devastated the rest of the world. I wonder what would've happened if Joseph hadn't refused to have sex with Potiphar's wife.

WRITE ABOUT IT

Q: In what ways do Joseph's choices apply to your own life?

the lust factor

THINK ABOUT IT

Q: Do you have a personal definition for lust?
  • How did you come to that definition?

Q: Where do you think lust begins? Why do you think that?
  • eye contact
  • touching arms
  • rubbing shoulders and backs
  • hugging
  • holding hands
  • prolonged hugging
  • cuddling
  • kiss on the cheek
  • kiss on the mouth
  • prolonged kissing
  • touching buttocks (clothed)
  • touching breasts or genitals (clothed)
  • rubbing bare skin underneath clothing
  • removing clothing
  • oral sex
  • intercourse

Q: How do you explain the fact that some people draw the line later than others?

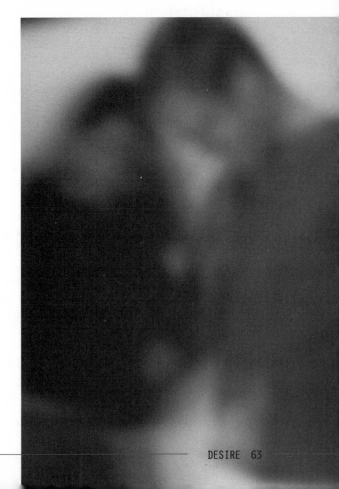

Q: What do you think is wrong with lust?

Look at Matthew 5:27-30.

Q: How do your thoughts about lust compare with this passage?

GOD'S-EYE VIEW

Matthew 5:28 is an unsettling answer to the question, "How far can I go?" I just want to know if I need to stop whatever I'm doing. Instead, Jesus tells me it's too late. I'm already guilty. In fact, I'm a repeat offender. Once again his answer is much bigger than my question.

WRITE ABOUT IT

Q: Are sexual lusts causing you trouble now?
   • If so, do you feed those lusts or starve them?
   • How do you feel about your answer?

is masturbation sex?

THINK ABOUT IT

Okay, so you've heard the word *masturbation* and maybe even joked about it with others in the school locker room. But do you really know what it means? Have you come to terms with what God might say about it—and with how God's opinion relates to your own behaviors?

Let's take one question at a time.

First, what is masturbation? That's pretty easy. It's touching your own genitals to stimulate yourself to orgasm.

Next, what does God say about it? Well, the word *masturbation* never appears in the Bible. Some Christians believe masturbation is always wrong, for these reasons. First, it often involves visualizing someone of the opposite gender—someone you're not married to, which they would oppose. Second, it's a form of sexual stimulation, and sexual stimulation should be saved for marriage. Others believe it's perfectly fine and normal because teens as well as adults can use it as a way to release sexual pressures that build up inside of them. Still others fall somewhere in the middle and say that it may be okay at times, but it can easily become addictive and controlling, so do it only rarely.

> Of a surveyed group of men, 71 percent who have been exposed to pornography felt that it degraded sex; 80 percent felt it was degrading to women; 97 percent felt it was harmful.
> —from a survey by Archibald D. Hart, in The Sexual Man (Word Books,

The problem is, most people find that once they start masturbating, they can't stop. Ron had that problem. He started masturbating in ninth grade because he was curious and it felt good. He did it more often in tenth grade, and pretty much every night in eleventh grade. Now that he's a senior, he's realizing it's starting to control him, and he wan to stop.

Well, at least part of him wants to stop. Another part of him enjoys it and wants to do it even more.

So Ron's really confused. He's tried everything he's heard of that might help—taking cold showers, exercising, avoiding any pictures of girls that might get him thinking about sex—but still he feels trapped.

Q: What would you say to Ron if he asked you what he should do?

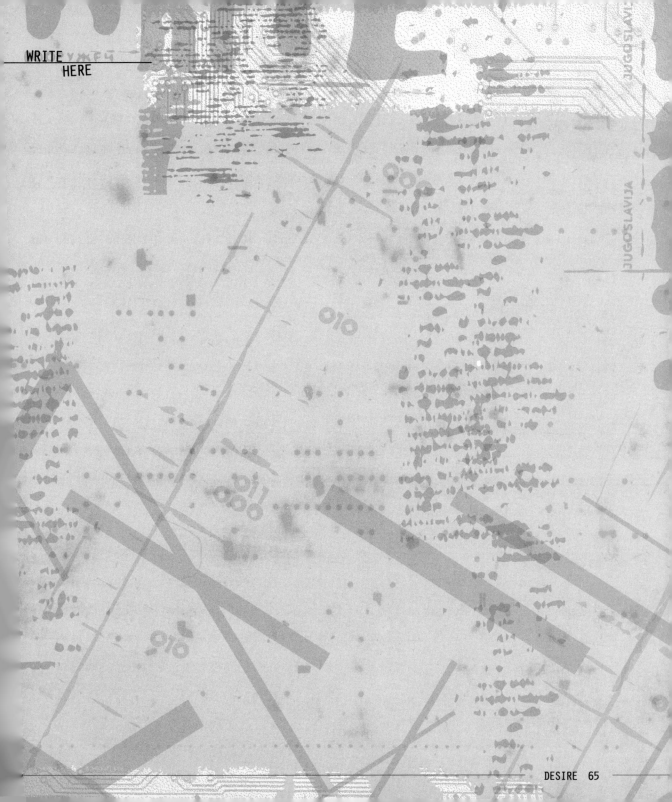

Q: How does I Corinthians 10:13 relate to masturbation?

Let's keep looking through the Bible. Find James 1:12-15. We've used it in other parts of this book, but it sure fits here.

Q: How could masturbation become a temptation that results in sin?
 • Do you think it's possible to masturbate only occasionally—unlike Ron, who found it addictive and controlling?

Q: Okay, now let's get more personal. Forget Ron. Given I Corinthians 10:13 and James 1:12-15, how do you think God would want *you* to act when it comes to masturbation?

> No temptation has seized you except what is common to man. And God is faithful; he will not let you be tempted beyond what you can bear. But when you are tempted, he will also provide a way out so that you can stand up under it.   I Corinthians 10:13

are you coming on to me

WRITE ABOUT IT

Q: List as many signals as you can think of that someone is coming on to you.

Q: How can you tell if someone welcomes your advances?
 • How can you tell if they don't?
 • How do you feel when someone doesn't seem to welcome your flirting or more sincere advances? What do you think this says about you?
Q: If you've had any bad experiences with flirting or coming on to someone, what did you learn in the process?
 • Did that change your behavior?
 • Could you use some help in learning to express your attraction to others without flirting?

write here

WRITE HERE

WRITE HERE

BOUNDARIES 5

The Bible doesn't acknowledge the one question unmarried people most often ask—at least not directly. The question goes something like this.

I know I'm not supposed to have sex, okay? But how far can I go? Second base? Third base?

You may not like the answer. Because the Bible doesn't really talk about sexluv&dating in any modern sense. What the Bible does talk about—quite a bit, actually—is lust.

So here it is:

You can go as far as you want—as long as you stop before you lust.

Lust is a serious fixation on something that's not ours to have. It's a deep, focused, inappropriate craving. In the Bible, the images associated with lust are heavy breathing, smoldering, and bursting into flames. The Bible doesn't talk about hooking up—it talks about longing for experiences that are not rightly ours and breaking boundaries to get them.

This chapter is about learning to identify and respect sexual boundaries.

The trick is, not everybody lusts the same. Some people can hardly go to an art gallery or ballet without drooling, so forget about watching R-rated films and television. Some people are turned on by the least bit of exposed midriff, so that trip to the beach is going to be a problem. Some people can barely endure a hug, let alone a back rub, so youth group cuddling is out of the question. For those who lust easily, just being around other people is a trial, just turning on a computer is a temptation, just going to the pool (or beach or lake) is an ordeal.

Other folks have a much higher lust threshold—who knows why? They take in stride images and touch that drive other people crazy. Which is why Christians are called to a high level of sexual sensitivity. It's our duty to look out for each other and do our best to avoid tempting someone who may lust for different reasons than we do.

Turn over the coin. If your friends decide to ask each other, "What makes you lust?" then it's time to speak up for yourself. If sexual content in films and television is a problem for you, please say so. If short skirts drive you to distraction, please admit that. If brotherly hugs ignite un-sisterly fires in you, please sound off. And this is okay because you're not alone. We have different thresholds for lust, but sooner or later we all lust. Anyone who denies that simply hasn't gotten there yet, or they've decided to lie about it. It's just a matter of time.

the power of sex

THINK ABOUT IT

Look at Genesis 26:1-14.

Q: What do you think of Isaac's strategy to save his own life?
  • How do you imagine Rebekah felt about it?
  • Would you have gone along if you'd been in Rebekah's sandals?

Look again at Genesis 26:2-5.

Q: What do you think tipped off the king that Isaac and Rebekah weren't brother and sister?

GOD'S-EYE VIEW

The Hebrew word translated as *caressing* in the NIV actually means *playing*. The King James Version of the Bible uses the word *sporting*. It's a word that suggests intimate giggling. Whatever they were giggling about when the king looked out his window was something he knew a healthy guy doesn't do with his sister.

Q: Do you think Isaac really loved Rebekah? What makes you think that?
  • How do you explain Isaac's choice to expose Rebekah to abuse?

Q: Why do you think sex has enough power that men would kill in order to be with women they have no right to be with?
  • Is it just me, or does it seem to you that women often get a raw deal when it comes to sex?

what ivory soap has to do with sex

THINK ABOUT IT

You'd think most of this would go without saying, but maybe not. Look at Leviticus 20:7-24.

Q: Does anything here surprise you?

Q: What do you think the word *consecrate* means?

GOD'S-EYE VIEW

In Leviticus 20:7, *consecration* means people exercise their will to do God's will. Consecration is also an action to avoid contamination.

Q: What do you think the word *holy* means?

In Leviticus 20:7, holiness is purity. To be holy is to be all one thing, unadulterated by anything else. As they used to say a while ago, "Ivory soap is 99 and 44/100ths percent pure," which is pretty clean, but not quite holy.

Q: In verse 7, why do you think God calls for consecration and holiness?
   • In verse 8, what part does God claim to play in our holiness?
   • If this is the case, what part do you think we play in our own holiness?

Q: This is a long list of no-nos. What reasons does God give for prohibiting these behaviors?

Q: Do you suppose if something isn't on this list, that means it's okay?

Q: How do you account for the harshness of the penalty for these acts? (I mean, "kill them" is not exactly the same as "get them in a 12-step group.")

GOD'S-EYE VIEW

Look at John 8:1-11. As you read John 8 and compare it with Leviticus 20, the issue of the relationship between the Old Testament and New Testament becomes pretty obvious. The New Testament doesn't make the teachings of the Old Testament void. Rather the death and resurrection of Jesus provides a new, ultimate way for us humans to experience God's forgiveness. Since Jesus is the ultimate sacrifice for sin, we no longer have to sacrifice animals—or ourselves—when we sin (and boy, isn't that a great thing?). Instead, we can be purified and justified by repenting for all we've done wrong (see 1 John 1:9). And yet, as John 8 reveals, the forgiveness Jesus offers doesn't mean we have unlimited freedom to continue in our sinful patterns. As we experience his grace, we should be motivated by our own gratitude—and empowered by God—to change.

Q: How does this story in the book of John compare to Leviticus 20?
   • What is similar between the two?
   • How are the two different?

Q: The woman appears to have been caught right in the act—which, as you may be aware, takes two people. Why do you suppose they brought the woman to Jesus, but not the man?

yes, master

THINK ABOUT IT

Look at 1 Corinthians 5:1-13.

Q: What seems to be the problem Paul is concerned with in the first few verses?

Paul seems to be arguing that one bad apple can spoil the barrel. A little yeast changes the whole lump of dough. He's concerned that the church at Corinth is being badly influenced because some guy is sleeping with his stepmother and no one seems to care. In fact, they seem to think it's a good thing.

WRITE ABOUT IT

Look at 1 Corinthians 6:9-11.

Q: What strikes you as the big idea in verses 9-11?
 • What seems surprising in these verses?

GOD'S-EYE VIEW

Washing is a complete cleansing. *Sanctification* is to be made holy. And *justification* is to be made innocent.

The culture of Corinth was divided into two major schools of thought about the human body. One side believed the human body was so worthless it ought to be thrashed and starved into submission—not a widely popular point of view. The other side believed the body was of little importance compared to the spirit, so they compartmentalized people into body and spirit—separate parts that didn't have much to do with each other. This school of thought figured there was no reason to deny the body anything it craved since the body was destined to go away anyhow and the real self was located in the spirit. In the next verses, Paul takes on those arguments and turns them inside out.

WRITE ABOUT IT

Look at 1 Corinthians 6:12-20.

Q: What do you think Paul is saying about food and sex?

Q: Given 1 Corinthians 6:16-17, what's the difference between being one with your spouse and one with someone who's not your spouse? Why is that?

The word *unite* comes from the image of gluing together, so 1 Corinthians 6:17 could easily be translated, "The one who glues herself to the Lord is one with him in spirit."

THINK ABOUT IT

Q: What do you think it means to flee from sexual immorality?
 • Do you believe that's more difficult at some times than at others?

Q: Do you believe sexual wrongs are different from other wrongs?
 • Do you believe God believes sexual wrongs are more wrong than other sins?

Q: How do you feel about the big payoff in 1 Corinthians 6:19-20, which reads, "You are not your own; you were bought at a price. Therefore honor God with your body"?
- What do you think he means when he says you were bought at a price? What price?
- What do you think it means to honor God with your body?
- And what do you think that person might get in return?
- Do you think it's worth it?

when is it sex?

WRITE ABOUT IT

When do you think it's sex? Identify the behavior you think is the threshold of sex between two people and explain your reasons.

- ❏ "I'll show you mine if you'll show me yours" because—
- ❏ Hugging because—
- ❏ Hand-holding because—
- ❏ Massaging because—
- ❏ Kissing because—
- ❏ Caressing because—
- ❏ Mutual masturbation because—
- ❏ Oral sex because—
- ❏ Sexual intercourse because—

Q: How did you reach that conclusion?

Q: Did we leave out anything you think should be on the list?

Q: List as many reasons as you can for delaying sexual intercourse until marriage.
- List as many reasons as you can for having sex early and often.

Q: Which reasons are most convincing to you? What makes them persuasive?

GOD'S-EYE VIEW

The Bible has all sorts of things to say about sex—but to be honest, it never gives an exact answer about the age-

WRITE HERE

old question *How far is too far?* Instead, it gives us guidelines to help us figure it out. Take I Thessalonians 4:3-5, where Paul says this:

> **It is God's will that you should be sanctified: that you should avoid sexual immorality; that each of you should learn to control his own body in a way that is holy and honorable, not in passionate lust like the heathen, who do not know God.**

WRITE ABOUT IT

Q: What do you think it means to control your body in a way that's holy?
  • If you were to do what you just wrote, how far would you go sexually with someone?

Q: Let's put it another way. Imagine you are a parent of a teenager your age who asks you how far he or she can go sexually. What would you say?

mother may i?

WRITE ABOUT IT

These people want to have sex, and they're looking for your approval. Check yes or no and give your reason.

• She's going to war—she may not come home alive. May I?

  ❑ Yes   ❑ No
  Because—

• He has cancer—we don't know if they caught it in time. May I?

  ❑ Yes   ❑ No
  Because—

• We're going to be married in less than a year. May I?

  ❑ Yes   ❑ No
  Because—

• We're going to be married in less than a week. May I?

  ❑ Yes   ❑ No
  Because—

• But I really, really love him—I'm afraid he may not wait. May I?

  ❑ Yes   ❑ No
  Because—

Q: Are you wishing you had special permission these days? Why?
  • What do you plan to do about that?
  • Who can help you work your way through this desire?

Q: Do you think God gives you special permission? Why or why not? If you're not sure, look up Proverbs 1:10, Proverbs 7:1-27, Romans 6:12-14, and 1 Peter 2:9.

~~what difference~~ does it make?

Q: If you think it makes a difference to save sex for marriage, say so—and give your reason.

  • I've done everything else. At this point it's just a technicality. What difference does it make?
    I think it makes a difference because—

  • I already did it with people I dated before I was a Christian. What difference does it make?
    I think it makes a difference because—

  • We've been doing it almost as long as we've been dating. It's too late to turn back. What difference does it make?
    I think it makes a difference because—

  • My mother does it with her boyfriend. And I know she expects me to do it too because she left a package of condoms on my bed—that tells you what she thinks of me. So what difference does it make?
    I think it makes a difference because—

  • I'm afraid Jesus will come back before I have sex, and I'll miss it. Besides, I know God will forgive me. I mean, he has to—he's God. I mean really, what difference does it make?
    I think it makes a difference because—

  • I was raped by my stepbrother, okay? And I feel like a piece of garbage. So what difference does it make?
    I think it makes a difference because—

Q: Do you think what you do sexually matters today? Why?

being "careful"

A few months after his prom night, my friend Jim told me what it was like for him to have sex for the first time:

I guess there wasn't really a moment when I decided, but it was like a process of decisions leading up to it. I'd been going out with this girl for a few weeks. Our physical relationship got way ahead of everything else—we hardly even talked sometimes. I figured sex might just happen, if the night was good enough—and prom night is usually kind of special.

I knew I needed to be careful so I bought my first condoms. So that was a big step for me, I guess. And when it finally came down to it, it was kind of clinical, actually—there were so many more factors that went through my head. I needed to find a place and a time. A place where we could get alone and no one would find out. It ended up being some kind of an operation, where I had to take care of a whole bunch of logistical factors instead of just letting that moment I'd imagined take control.

I was really at odds with what I was believing and what I was doing. They were two totally different things.

THINK ABOUT IT

Q: What stands out for you about this story?

Q: What do you think of the argument that says, "If you can't be good, at least be careful"?
• What do you think God would say about it?

THINK ABOUT IT

If you think about the word *careful*, it basically means *being full of care*. It's too bad that when it comes to sex, being "careful" has been reduced to making sure you use condoms—when in reality, being careful should mean being full of care for the people involved in your sexual decisions, meaning yourself and the other person. (Oh, and God!)

And here's a mind-blowing thought. What if you based your sexual actions on what was best and most caring for your future spouse? How might that affect the sexual boundaries you create for yourself?

i was drunk

I've had friends who used alcohol as an excuse to go farther than they said they would go. Others were taken where nobody wants to go because they were drunk.

"I had too much to drink," they say. "I'm not sure how it happened."

I've even heard friends say, "I'm not sure what happened. I hope I didn't do anything bad."

One friend was raped by several boys at a party while she was under the influence. She woke up the next morning sore and hung over. When she realized what had happened the night before, she freaked out and spent several days in a psychiatric hospital. It's been hard for her to come back from that experience.

Another girl was also attacked. She was sober enough to fight off the boy who climbed on top of her, but my other friend was too far gone to defend herself. They were both so ashamed and afraid of getting in trouble with their parents that they never told anybody. Well, that's not quite true. My friend told me this story from her hospital bed after narrowly surviving a suicide attempt. This most serious attempt on her life came after several years of bulimia and sexual craziness. It was another half decade before she started to live a normal life.

Sometimes I wonder what it is that makes some people prefer to not know—or not seem to know—what they're doing sexually. And what is it about alcohol that can put people in a position where they can't defend themselves?

THINK ABOUT IT

Q: Any of those stories sound familiar to you?

Q: What do you think is going on with girls (or boys) who use alcohol to set each other up sexually?

Q: Have you ever seen that work out well for anyone?

Look at Romans 13:9-14.

Q: How do you think this passage applies to the "I was drunk" excuse?

write here

RESPONSIBILITY

6

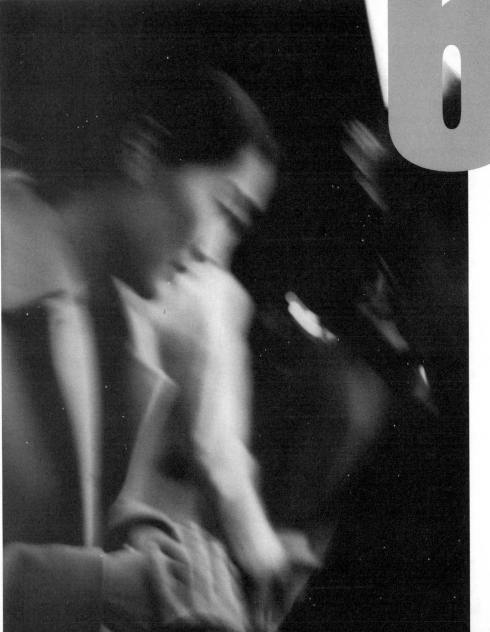

RESPONSIBILITY

Like it or not, we're all responsible for our own sexual behavior. Acting as if it were true—actually taking responsibility—is what this chapter is about.

It's like the rules of the road. Every state has some version of the Basic Speed Law, which states that motorists may drive only as fast as is reasonable under prevailing conditions. That means drivers must slow down on wet or slippery pavement, regardless of the posted speed limit and no matter what others do. "Everyone else was driving 65" is interesting but doesn't get you out of trouble if you skid into a car on a slick highway. You still get the moving violation. And if you're lucky, that's all you get.

"Everybody does it" is no excuse for behavior that violates the Basic Speed Law of sexuality. You're not responsible for everybody else, but you are responsible for yourself.

It's not hard to understand sexual responsibility. Just ask, "What are the prevailing conditions of my life? And given these conditions, what is responsible sexual behavior?"

"Yeah, but you don't understand my situation. I'm not a slut or anything—maybe I'm just hornier than most people."

That's an interesting theory, but if someone gets hurt, you're still responsible for your behavior.

"No, but you don't understand—my girlfriend is really hot. I can't control myself."

Sorry, but if you lose control, that means you're driving too fast for prevailing conditions.

"But, seriously, I think about sex all the time. That *is* my prevailing condition. Why would God give me hormonal urges and then tell me not to fulfill them? That's just mean."

It's not mean. It's a measure of human responsibility. If we were animals, we'd just satisfy our urges. We're not. Humans are all that and a bag of chips. We have the capacity to live above our basic instincts, to live sacrificially, to live heroically.

About now you may be saying, "Fine, I'm responsible. Tell me to whom and for what, and I'll give it a shot."
Fair enough.

- We're responsible to God, because God made us and we belong to God before we belong to ourselves or anybody else.

- We're responsible to each other, because we are brothers and sisters before we are anything else on the earth.

- We're responsible to ourselves, because even if we don't understand it, that inexpressible longing we feel is the longing to become what God made us to become.

Read what the apostle Paul says about it.

"It is God's will that you should be sanctified: that you should avoid sexual immorality; that each of you should learn to control his own body in a way that is holy and honorable, not in passionate lust like the heathen, who do not know God; and that in this matter no one should wrong his brother or take advantage of him. The Lord will punish men for all such sins, as we have already told you and warned you. For God did not call us to be impure, but to live a holy life" (1 Thessalonians 4:3-7).

Paul's definition of sanctification here is avoiding sexual immorality, learning to control our bodies in a way that's holy and honorable, and doing no harm to our sisters and brothers. And you may not have to look outside your own youth group to see out-of-control people taking advantage of their brothers or sisters in Christ. Pity.

Paul spins it another way in a letter to the church at Rome.

"Let us behave decently, as in the daytime, not in orgies and drunkenness, not in sexual immorality and debauchery, not in dissension and jealousy. Rather, clothe yourselves with the Lord Jesus Christ, and do not think about how to gratify the desires of the sinful nature" (Romans 13:13-14).

It's a vivid image. People who put on Christ have a fighting chance at thinking about more than just how to gratify their own desires. For people who aren't clothed with Jesus, it's an uphill battle.

A lot of people lose that fight just about every day. Maybe you're one of them. Maybe you live in an endless spiral of determination, failure, resolution, failure, recommitment, failure, remorse, failure—all because you think clothing yourself with the Lord Jesus Christ means asking, "What would Jesus do?" and then attempting to behave as decently as you can—which, it turns out, is not all that decent. It's not that you're worse than other people, it's just that, as Jesus put it, "apart from me, you can do nothing." In that line of reasoning, it takes more than good intentions to power good behavior.

If you're going to win the fight, your only hope is to ask Jesus to help you win it. That takes a more thorough conversion than many have yet experienced.

But then you need to ask others to help you also. Along with a deepening intimacy with the God who alone can sanctify you and make you holy, acting responsibly takes support and accountability in the community of God's people.

what's most important?

GOD'S-EYE VIEW

In Jesus' time, Jewish teachers had identified 613 statutes or commandments to obey. Of these 613 commandments, 365 were negative (meaning things people shouldn't do) and 248 were positive (meaning things people should do).

Look at Mark 12:28-31.

Q: Jesus' use of the word *all* (or *holos*, in Greek [HAUL'-oss]) means *altogether, every bit.* Do you think it's possible to love God with all of you? Why or why not?
 • How about loving your neighbor as yourself? Do you think that's possible? Why?

Q: Realize for a moment that God loves you. How does that influence your ability to love him back?

Q: Given the love God has shown you, and the love he wants you to show him, does that obligate you to behave in certain ways? Let's get even more specific: does that make you responsible to him for your sexual choices? Reflect on that a bit.

WRITE HERE

WRITE HERE WRITE HERE

Look at Galatians 6:1-2.

Q: Do you think this relates to the subject we're talking about? Why or why not?
  • How do you suppose we would treat others sexually if we viewed them as brothers or sisters in Christ even more than we viewed them as dating partners?
  • If we're treating dating partners primarily as brothers or sisters in Christ, what would some of our responsibilities be toward them?

u da man!

THINK ABOUT IT

Look at 2 Samuel 12:1-25.

Q: What do you think about David's reaction to the story? Is it about right under the circumstances? Too much? Why do you say that?

GOD'S-EYE VIEW

The interesting thing is that Nathan worked through the whole process with David. He didn't just confront David and then abandon him. He stuck around to celebrate the gift of David and Bathsheba's second son, Solomon.

Q: Put yourself back in Nathan's shoes. You've been sent to the king with the word that Solomon, his new baby, should also be known as *Jedidiah*, which means *Beloved of God*. This one is loved by the God of the universe. How do you think you would feel about bringing that message?
  • Think for a moment—has God already sent someone who brought you a message regarding something you need to change?
  • If so, what happened?

WRITE ABOUT IT

Look at Matthew 5:27-28.

Q: Does this passage speak to your situation today?

Q: Is there a Christian you know who's in sexual trouble?
  • If so, do you think there's any chance God may want you to play the part of Nathan for that person?
  • If so, what are you going to do about it?

excuses, excuses

GOD'S-EYE VIEW

Here's some background.

When the Lord destroyed Sodom and Gomorrah in Genesis 19, he promised to protect Lot in the city of Zoar. After Lot's two sons-in-law refused to leave Sodom and his wife looked back at the destruction of the city and turned into a pillar of salt, he and his two daughters were the only members of his family to escape.

Genesis 13:5-6 says Lot had so many possessions that the land where he lived with his uncle Abraham wouldn't support them all. (Which is why Lot ended up moving to Sodom to begin with.) Contrast that with his situation in Genesis 19:30 where he's reduced to living in a cave—though it was probably a very nice cave.

THINK ABOUT IT

Look at Genesis 19:30-36.

Q: Although in verse 30, God promised Lot safety in the city of Zoar, he left Zoar and hid in a cave. What do you think that says about Lot's trust in God?

Q: What reasons does the older daughter give for sleeping with her dad? What do you think of her reasons?

Look at Genesis 19:6-11 and 15-16.

Q: Given that Lot's daughters were rescued from the mob in Sodom in Genesis 19:6-11, and then rescued from the destruction of Sodom in verses 15 and 16, what do their actions tell you about their trust in God?

WRITE ABOUT IT

Q: How have you seen your friends take advantage of someone sexually or emotionally?
   • What are the consequences for a person who gets taken advantage of sexually or emotionally?
   • How about for the person who takes advantage—do you believe there are consequences for that person?
   • If they are both part of the same Christian community, what consequences do you think it can have on the body of Christ? Why?

entitlement

Most people cross back and forth across the line between entitlement and servanthood.

   • *Entitlement*—I should get whatever I want whenever I want it. (For example, if I want to lust after a woman's body, I'll go ahead and do that. If I want to cheat on my boyfriend, I'll do it.)
   • *Servanthood*—I'll look out for the interests of others, even when it costs me. (For example, since lusting after a woman's chest can hurt both her and me, I'll use self-control and won't do it. If cheating on my boyfriend can hurt us both, I'll control myself and forget about it.)

Read the following stories and consider where these individuals fall on the line between entitlement and servanthood.

> Robyn has a great body, and she sure knows how to show it off. She always wears these short, tight skirts and skimpy tank tops. Unless, of course, it's cold, in which case she wears skintight pants and a form-fitting sweater. Since math class is arranged alphabetically, Jon sits right next to Robyn. When Robyn walks into the room, Jon can't help but notice that she's wearing a tight denim skirt and a revealing pink T-shirt. A few minutes later, as Robyn turns sideways in her seat, Jon is having a hard time keeping his mind on his algebra. His eyes really want to wander—and maybe stay to enjoy the view. Suddenly Jon hears someone asking, "What are you looking at?" Glancing up, he realizes it's Robyn, and she's looking right at him.

THINK ABOUT IT

Q: Do you think Robyn is expressing entitlement?

Q: Do you think Jon is expressing entitlement?

Q: How do you think Robyn could express servanthood?

Q: How do you think Jon could express servanthood?

> Blanca can't wait for winter formal. She just knows that Billy—a guy in her PE class who always just happens to end up on the same team with her—will invite her. When she finds a note in her locker, her heart starts pounding and her hands start sweating. It's an invitation to the dance.
>
> When she reads the end of the note, her excitement evaporates. It's signed "Eric Lopez," not "Billy Abbiate." She knows she'll see Eric in English after lunch, so she has less than an hour to figure out what to do.

Q: How do you think Blanca could express entitlement?

Q: How do you think Blanca could express servanthood?

Q: What do you think you would do in Blanca's situation? Why?

> Danny's in the kitchen making root beer floats for three friends who are spending the night. When he walks back into the family room with a tray full of glasses, napkins, and massive doses of sugar, all three friends are huddled around his computer. Philip is downloading images from a pornography site, and while Max seems really into it, Aaron looks uneasy. All four boys go to the same church. Max and Philip are sophomores. Danny and Aaron, who are seniors, kind of want to take Max and Philip under their wing. Now they're not sure what to do.

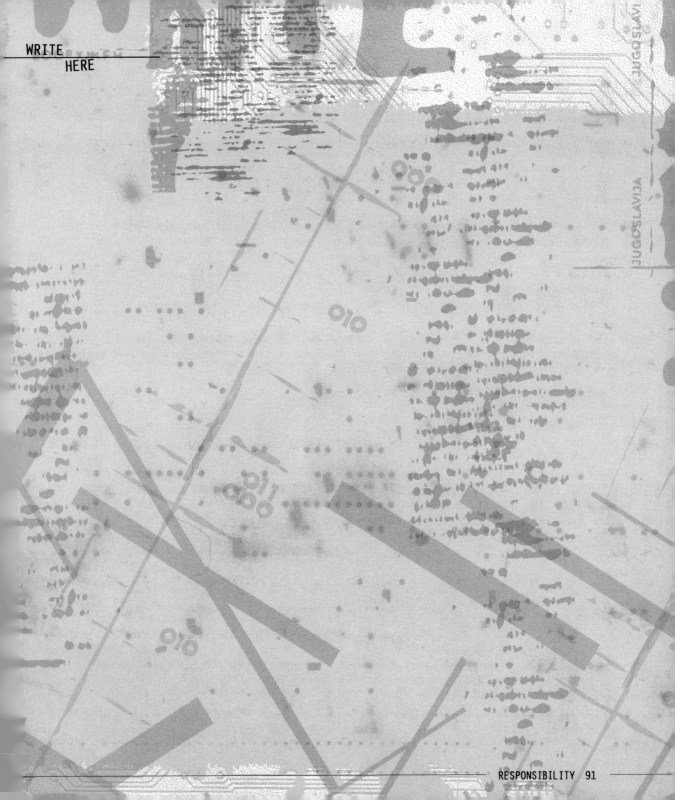

WRITE
HERE

Q: How do you think Danny and Aaron could express entitlement?

Q: How do you think Philip and Max could express entitlement?

Q: How do you think Danny and Aaron could express servanthood?

Q: How do you think Philip and Max could express servanthood?

> Whoever wants to be first must be your slave—just as the Son of Man did not come to be served, but to serve, and to give his life as a ransom for many.
>
> —Jesus, speaking to his disciples in Matthew 20:27-28

WRITE ABOUT IT

Q: How do you think your life would be different if you were 100 percent oriented toward entitlement? Why?
• What would change if you were 100 percent oriented toward servanthood? Please be as specific as you can.

Q: What difference would a servant attitude make in the way you look at—and I mean that literally, *look at*—members of the opposite gender? Why is that?
• What difference do you think a servant attitude would make in the way you treat them? Why?

Q: What do you think it would take for you to stay in servant mode 100 percent of the time?
• Is there someone you can ask to help you with that? If not, is there someone you ask to help you with the fact that there's no one you can turn to for support?

this is a test

WRITE ABOUT IT

Q1: What percentage of Americans over the age of 11 show evidence of genital herpes?

Q2: What percentage of sexually transmitted infections occur in people under the age of 25?

Q3: What percentage of girls who get pregnant before age 18 earn a high school diploma by the age of 30?

Q4: What percentage of Americans are infected with HIV?

Q5: What percentage of women infected by chlamydia don't know they're infected because they have no obvious symptoms?

Q6: What percentage of men infected by chlamydia don't know they're infected because they have no obvious symptoms?

Q7: What percentage of people infected by chlamydia (who don't know they're infected because they have no obvious symptoms) are capable of infecting another person with the disease?

Q8: What percentage of people using condoms for contraception become pregnant within the first year of use?

Q9: What percentage of adolescents who have had sexual intercourse are no longer sexually active?

Q10: What percentage of American males and females ages 15 to 19 are still virgins?

Check your answers.

Q1: More than 20 percent—that's about one in five—of Americans over the age of 11 show evidence of genital herpes.

Q2: About 66 percent—that's about two out of three—sexually transmitted infections occur in people under the age of 25.

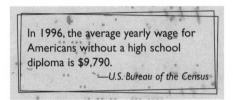

In 1996, the average yearly wage for Americans without a high school diploma is $9,790.

—U.S. Bureau of the Census

Q3: 30 percent of women—seven of 10—don't get a high school diploma by age 30 if pregnant before age 18.

Q4: About .003 percent of Americans—that's three of every 10,000—are infected with HIV.

Q5: Up to 85 percent of women infected by chlamydia—that's almost nine out of 10—don't know they're infected because they have no obvious symptoms.

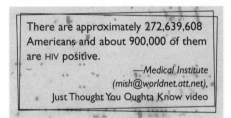

There are approximately 272,639,608 Americans and about 900,000 of them are HIV positive.

—Medical Institute
(mish@worldnet.att.net),
Just Thought You Oughta Know video

Q6: Up to 40 percent of men infected by chlamydia—that's four out of 10—don't know they're infected because they have no obvious symptoms.

Q7: 100 percent of people infected by chlamydia (who don't know they're infected because they have no obvious symptoms)—that would be 10 for 10 for those of you keeping score at home—are capable of infecting another person with the disease.

Q8: About 15 percent of people using condoms for contraception—more than one out of 10—become pregnant within the first year of use.

Q9: About 25 percent of adolescents who have had sexual intercourse—about one in four—stop soon after they start.

Q10: About 50 percent of American males and females ages 15 to 19—that's one in two—are still virgins.

Q: Do any of these percentages surprise you?

Q: Given this level of risk, if a person knows he's infected, what obligations do you think he has to anyone he dates? Why?
- What percentage of infected individuals do you believe live up to those obligations? Why do you think that?
- Do you know of anyone who's warned others that they are carriers of an infectious disease? What does that suggest to you?

Q: Do you know anyone who's gone for a blood test to see if they might be carriers of an STD? What does that suggest to you?

Q: Do you know anyone who might be infected by an STD?
- Do you believe that person might go for a blood test if you offered to go along? Why?

WRITE ABOUT IT

Q: If you've been sexually active, how do you know you're *not* infected?
- Have you been tested since your last sexual contact?

Q: What do you think is your responsibility to yourself and others when it comes to STDs? Why?

Q: Does the fear of contracting an STD make you not want to have sex again before you marry?

If you haven't had sex yet (and there's a 50 percent chance you haven't), how do STDs affect your sexual abstinence?

AIDS and HIV

THINK ABOUT IT

Q: Chances are, someone you know is infected with HIV. How do you feel about that?
- Are you aware of anyone who's infected?

Q: If you find out someone you know has AIDS, how do you think you should act toward that person? Why?
- What does it mean to act responsibly toward them?

Q: Do you have a different attitude toward people who get HIV or AIDS from homosexual behavior than people who get it from heterosexual contact or from a blood transfusion or other medical mishap? Why?

Q: How do you think Jesus would respond to a person with AIDS? Why? Maybe before you write your answer you should check out John 8:1-11.
- How do Jesus' final words in John 8:11 relate to how we should respond to people who have AIDS?

Q: If you learn that a friend has AIDS, what do you think you would do?

the home front

Q: What do you wish your parents understood about you and your dating life?
  • Why do you think people don't talk to their parents about dating and sex? Or is that just a stereotype?

Q: How comfortable are you talking with your parents about dating, love, or sex?

❑ Completely comfortable because—

❑ It depends because—

❑ Completely uncomfortable because—

  • How comfortable do your parents seem to feel talking with you about dating, love, or sex?

❑ Completely comfortable because—

❑ It depends because—

❑ Completely uncomfortable because—

Q: Do you believe that acting responsibly in your relationship with your parents means it's probably a good idea to talk with them about your life, including dating, love, or sex? Why or why not?

In Exodus 20:12, and then later in Ephesians 6:1-4, children are commanded to honor their parents.

Q: What does it mean to honor your parents? If you get stuck, think about what it means to "honor" someone at a banquet or surprise birthday party.
  • How do you think you can honor your parents in the middle of what you're experiencing emotionally and sexually?

write here

DO-OVERS

7

DO-OVERS

Sooner or later, everyone needs do-overs.

People who use sex as a weapon and people who've been hammered with sex. People who make bad choices and dumb mistakes. People whose sexual experiments blow up in their faces. People who know Mr. Lust is a born liar but believe him anyway (hey, maybe this time things will be different). People so arrogant or stupid they honestly think they're not like the rest of us. People consumed by thoughts of the next orgasm and people consumed with pride because they've never had sex. People who wish they knew back then what they know now—we know who we are.

Everybody, sooner or later, needs do-overs.

But can we get them?

Children learn about do-overs in friendly games of hopscotch or marbles. A do-over is a second chance when someone makes a mistake—it's a gift between friends. No one has a right to demand do-overs. No one can just say, "Shut up, I'm taking a do-over." A do-over is a favor, an act of grace. Grace is what this chapter is mainly about, do-overs for people who commit sexual fouls—that is to say, all of us.

First, the bad news. For single people, young and old, sex is a high-risk behavior, like driving under the influence. If nothing goes wrong, maybe nobody gets hurt. But if things go badly, maybe someone dies.

That worst-case scenario—someone dies—raises the stakes from, say, lying. Tell a lie, and if things go badly, the worst that happens (for you, at least) is you get caught and suffer the consequences of breaking trust. Unpleasant, but probably endurable.

> It's no secret that sex with the wrong person can be life-threatening.

Getting caught sexually includes outcomes like pregnancy and sexually transmitted diseases.

A solo pregnancy is endlessly difficult no matter what. Ask around—you may find women making the best of hard situations, but you'll be hard-pressed to find a single mother who thinks she got away with anything.

Ditto on sexually transmitted diseases. At this writing, half a dozen epidemics run amok in the sexually active population. They are presently unstoppable diseases for which there are treatments but no cure.

Don't think such things can happen to you? Please.

Getting caught sexually may also include unanticipated emotional consequences. There's an interesting idea in Paul's first letter to the Christians at Corinth. "Flee from sexual immorality," he says. "All other sins a man commits are outside his body, but he who sins sexually sins against his own body" (1 Corinthians 6:18). Sex has an unusually personal effect because it's uniquely inside rather than outside us—sex is not something we merely *do*.

This makes sense to those who've been surprised to find themselves feeling shame about things they didn't think were wrong when they did them. Some people respond to those feelings by building up calluses where the pain is, like the tough spots on a tennis player's hands or a dancer's feet. But a lot of people decide it's just not worth it. According to the Medical Institute for Sexual Health, one of every four adolescents who becomes sexually active stops soon after he or she begins. The good feelings they got from sex presumably didn't offset the bad feelings. The attachment they felt was nullified by the pain

DO-OVER

of separation. They gave it a shot, maybe more than one. But, eventually, it's like, why bother?

All of which begs the question: Can 16-year-old boys and girls burned out on premature sex get do-overs? The answer depends on how we answer another question: Is God for us or against us?

If God is against us, it's game over—there won't be any do-overs. We'll die forgiven but still guilty.

If, on the other hand, God is for us, there's hope. We still must contend with the natural consequences of our behavior, but there's supernatural hope. "There is," as Betsy ten Boom told her sister Corrie, "no pit so deep that God's love is not deeper still."

Just to be certain it's been said, let's underscore one lonely group of folk who need do-overs in spite of themselves. They are the ones who were—or, God forbid, are—abused by their fathers, brothers, sisters, uncles, aunts, cousins, babysitters, teachers, pastors, and boyfriends (if anyone's left out, it's only because it's too hard to go on).

These victims of sexualized violence—and it is violent, however silently it may creep—tend to blame and punish themselves for what was done *to* them (not *by* them).

~~a second, third,~~ and ~~sixty-third~~ chance

THINK ABOUT IT

Look at John 8:1-11.

Q: Put yourself on the edge of the crowd that morning. Someone comes in late and asks, "What's going on?" What would you tell them (other than, "Uh, I have to go now.")?

Q: If you were going strictly by the rules, does this passage leave any question that the woman was guilty?
- What about her accusers—does the story leave any doubt about their guilt?
- How does that idea fit the last thing Jesus says to the woman in this story, namely, "Go now and leave your life of sin" (John 8:11)?

WRITE ABOUT IT

Q: Does it feel more normal for you to treat people like Jesus treated the woman caught in the act of adultery or like her accusers treated people?

Q: Do you know anyone who's becoming a better person because he's getting sexual do-overs?

Q: Do you know someone who could use a sexual do-over now?

Q: And you? How easy is it for you to believe Jesus might really give you a do-over when you need one?

> To repent is to come to your senses. It is not so much something you do as something that happens. True repentance spends less time looking at the past and saying "I'm sorry," than looking at the future and saying, "Wow!"
>
> —*Frederick Buechner, Wishful Thinking: A Seeker's ABC (HarperCollins)*

Q: Given what Jesus said to the woman in John 8, what do you think he says to you—or anyone else for that matter—when you keep making the same mistake over and over again?

Q: Some people seem willing to sin over and over again because they know God will forgive them. Given Jesus' words in John 8, what do you think he would say about that?

falling...
and bouncing back

Before you read Psalms 32 and 51, review the story of David's great fall and recovery in 2 Samuel 11-12.

| WRITE ABOUT IT |

Look at 2 Samuel 11 and 12.

Q: What do you think David was feeling or thinking as these events unfolded? (Circle all that apply.)

lust	remorse	frustration	treachery
deceit	foolishness	arrogance	grief
hope	love	stupidity	guilt

calling your bluff

| THINK ABOUT IT |

Look at John 4:1-42.

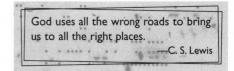

> God uses all the wrong roads to bring us to all the right places.
> —C. S. Lewis

Q: Why do you suppose Jesus struck up a conversation with this woman?

Q: What do you think about Jesus' choice of messengers for this town?

❑ She seems like an unlikely spokesperson for godliness because—

❑ She seems kinda right because—

❑ She seems perfect to me because—

Q: Have you ever seen God use this kind of messenger to reach people?

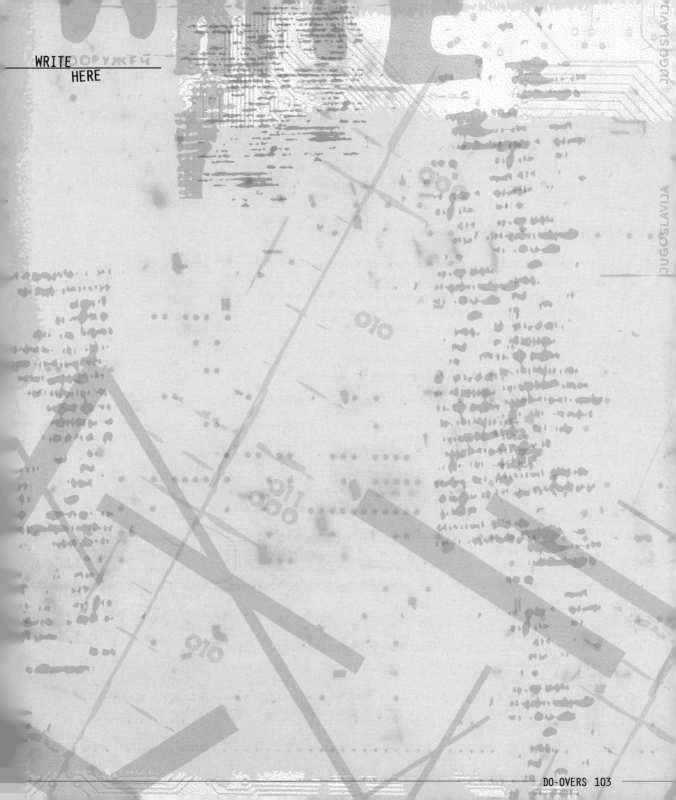

Q: Jesus called the woman's bluff when he asked her to bring her husband. Is there a question Jesus could ask you that would call your bluff?

WRITE ABOUT IT

Q: Would you consider what you've done (or failed to do) to be any worse (or better) than the woman in this story?

Q: Can you imagine using your story of failure to introduce people to Jesus? Why or why not?
  • What do you think you have to gain or lose by using your failure story to introduce people to Jesus? Is it worth it? Why?

From here, it looks like forgiven people come in two flavors:

  1. Those who feel so grateful to be forgiven that they stop judging other people and, like Jesus, become the friends of sinners.
  2. Those who feel they somehow deserved to be forgiven—some kind of exemption for special people, perhaps. They become very hard to live with because they're always pointing their fingers at people who do bad things or fail to do good things.

Q: Is it just me, or does it look that way to you as well?
  • Which kind of Christian do you want to hang with? Why?

welcome back...
or maybe not

GOD'S-EYE VIEW

Here's some background on 2 Corinthians 2:1-11, 7:8-12.
   In Paul's first letter to the Christians in the city of Corinth, he tells them to denounce a man who's sleeping with his mother-in-law. Refer to the Bible study on this subject (pages 73, 75). There's no specific record of how the church responded, but apparently it caused quite a stir because Paul's follow-up letter goes further into the episode.

THINK ABOUT IT

Q: What strikes you as the most significant thing Paul says in these two passages?
  • Why do you think that's significant?

Q: Paul seems to believe that a private act (a man sleeping with his father's wife) has community consequences (2 Corinthians 2:5). Have you ever seen that connection played out within a Christian group?
  • If so, what did you observe?

WRITE HERE

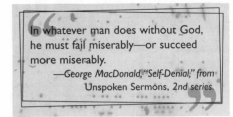

WRITE ABOUT IT

Q: From what Paul says about this episode in the life of the Corinthian church, how do you imagine Paul viewed sexual wrongdoing?

- ❏ Less serious than other wrongs because—

- ❏ The same as other wrongs because—

- ❏ More serious than other wrongs because—

Q: How do Paul's words change your own attitude about sexual wrongs?

scarlet ~~lady~~

Look at Joshua 1-6, Hebrews 11:31, and James 2:25.

THINK ABOUT IT

Q: What do you think is the most important thing that comes out of Rahab's story? Why do you think that's important?

Q: Why do you think God works with people like Rahab? Why not a queen or a Joan of Arc type?

WRITE ABOUT IT

Look at 1 Corinthians 1:26-31.

Q: Comparing this passage to Joshua 1-6, Hebrews 11:31, and James 2:25, what do you learn about God?
- Why do you think that picture of God stands out for you?

Q: Are there any ways that you're like Rahab? If so, how?
- Are there ways in which God is treating you like he treated Rahab? How?

Q: If this is true about how God accepts people, what do you want to do in response?

you want me to marry a what?

A bit of background on Hosea 1-3—

Anytime you read Hosea 1-3, it's important to remember that Hosea was a prophet who included his own life story as part of the message God has for his people. Just as Hosea took Gomer back even when she had been unfaithful, God was willing to take the Israelites back even after they had worshiped other gods.

THINK ABOUT IT

Look at Hosea 1-3.

WRITE ABOUT IT

Q: If you were Hosea's friend, and he told you what he thought God was asking him to do, what would you have told him? Why?
  • If you were Gomer's friend, and she told you she was going to marry the prophet, what would you have told her?

Q: Now imagine that God is in the place of Hosea, and you are in the place of Gomer. Whether or not you've had an affair, there are all sorts of other ways you've chosen to turn your back on God. Given Hosea's actions (remembering that Hosea represents God), what do you think God would say to you about your own sin and disobedience against him?
  • What two or three things could you do that would help you better serve and love God this month?

Jesus, the unexpected

THINK ABOUT IT

Look at Luke 7:36-50.

Q: With whom do you most identify in this story?

❏ Simon the Pharisee because—

❏ The woman because—

❏ Jesus because—

❏ The other guests because—

WRITE
HERE

Q: How long do you think Jesus would last on the staff of a local church or Christian organization? Why?

Q: How long do you think it would take the woman in this story to fit in at that local church? Why?

Q: Do you think most Christians really believe Jesus when he says things like he said about (and to) this woman?

Q: Do you think people have to be prostitutes to appreciate how much they've been forgiven?

WRITE ABOUT IT

Q: How well do you do at treating people as if Jesus is really serious about ministry to outcasts?

❑ Not well at all because—

❑ I could do better because—

❑ I could do worse because—

❑ Pretty well most of the time because—

Q: What do you think you may have yet to really learn from this story? Write a note to God about that.

write here

WRITE
HERE

Plumbing and Wiring:
FAQs

We're just trying to respond honestly to the questions teens ask. So skip the ones you think are obvious and just be glad there's somebody out there who knows less than you. Feel free to circle whether you knew it or didn't.

Q: How do people learn to kiss?
The truth is that kissing comes pretty naturally to a girl and a guy. Sometimes noses get bumped and braces get locked up, but those mishaps are rare.
knew it/didn't know it

Q: How do people breathe when they kiss?
Although girls' and guys' mouths are pretty preoccupied during kissing, their noses usually aren't—they do the work for them.
knew it/didn't know it

Q: What exactly happens during sex?
The sexual act proceeds through several phases. The first is an excitement phase, marked by an increase in pulse and blood pressure as blood rushes to the surface of the body. Genital fluids are also secreted during the excitement phase. The penis becomes erect, and the vagina expands. The second phase is the plateau phase, which is pretty brief and may conclude with an orgasm. The third phase is the resolution phase where the body functions return to normal.
knew it/didn't know it

Q: What is an orgasm?
An orgasm, also called a *climax*, is the peak of physical sexual excitement and gratification. Physically, it's marked by a faster pulse, higher blood pressure, and muscle contractions in the penis and vagina. Sperm ejaculates from the penis. An orgasm is marked by an overwhelming feeling of pleasure and release.
knew it/didn't know it

Q: Does an orgasm always happen during intercourse?
Not always. Sometimes two people will feel fairly aroused and have a grand ol' time together, but neither will have an orgasm. It's also possible to have an orgasm before or after sexual intercourse.
knew it/didn't know it

Q: Is an orgasm different for a guy than for a girl?

Well, yes, because they have different body parts. Both experience quick, rapid muscular contractions, but the female's orgasm usually lasts longer. Another bonus for the female is that she can often have several orgasms in succession, while the male usually has one. However, one bonus for the male is that since he usually becomes more quickly aroused, he has orgasms more consistently during sexual intercourse.

knew it/didn't know it

Q: Do orgasms always feel the same?

No, an orgasm almost always feels good, but sometimes it feels great. How great relates to how emotionally connected you are to the other person, how physically tired and aroused you are, how mentally distracted you are, and how comfortable you feel to enjoy what's going on.

knew it/didn't know it

Q: How long does an orgasm last?

Although the orgasm is the most talked-about phase in sexual intercourse, it's actually short, ranging from five to 30 seconds.

knew it/didn't know it

Q: What's an erection?

When a male becomes sexually aroused, the blood flow into his penis is increased and the blood flowing out of his penis is temporarily reduced. As a result, the tissue swells, and the penis enlarges, hardens, and elevates.

knew it/didn't know it

> I used to think I would just want to have sex 24 hours a day. I didn't know that the body parts just get tired and sore after a while. I didn't know that sometimes I would just be too tired to care about it and just want to go to sleep.
>
> —*Hanna, on the information she got about sex*

Q: I've heard that alcohol will help your sex drive, but I've also heard it will hurt it. What's the deal?

Alcohol is a depressant, so it tends to reduce inhibitions and dull decision-making skills. So people who've had something to drink may become more flirtatious or willing to try things they wouldn't even consider when sober. Because of this, some people jump to the conclusion that alcohol increases sex drive. But actually alcohol depresses the nervous system and diminishes muscular coordination and nerve sensation. Sober sex is generally more pleasurable than sex under the influence. Perhaps the biggest gotcha is that the risk of pregnancy and contracting sexually transmitted infections increases with carelessness, so reread the first sentence and do the math.

knew it/didn't know it

Q: Does sex hurt?

It can hurt—especially the first few times and especially for women. Imagine going dancing for the first time. Since you don't know what you're doing—and you haven't practiced—you might hurt yourself or the other person. The same is true for sex when you're new at it. This is one reason your patient, caring, committed partner (by which we mean *spouse*) can make the experience go more smoothly. This is especially true when you both believe practice makes perfect.
knew it/didn't know it

Q: Does the size of the penis matter?

Most males assume the average size of an erect penis is 6 inches, and then they get worried because theirs is smaller than that. But the reality is that an erect penis measures around 5.1 to 5.2 inches, and a nonerect (or flaccid) penis measures 3.5 inches. Regardless of the penis size, the male doesn't need to worry about it. The female's body adjusts to fit whatever size he is.
knew it/didn't know it

Q: Is masturbation wrong?

Ah, that's a biggie. Masturbation, or stimulating your own genitals, is pretty controversial. Some Christians believe it's wrong all the time, others believe it's right almost all of the time—and still others fall somewhere in the middle, arguing that it's okay to do periodically as long as it isn't associated with lustful fantansies or doesn't become a preoccupation (which it tends to become the more you do it). You might want to talk to a parent or Christian adult you respect to get some more guidance. There's more about masturbation in **Desire** (page 64).
knew it/didn't know it

Q: What is oral sex?

Contrary to what some may think, *oral* sex is not *talking about* sex. Instead, it means using the mouth to stimulate another person's genitals.
knew it/didn't know it

Q: Is oral sex the same as sex?

By definition, no (in the sense that babies can't be born from oral sex). But don't forget that sexually transmitted infections can be contracted through oral sex and that it's way past the line of what you want to be doing before marriage.
knew it/didn't know it .

Q: What if my breasts are different sizes?

That's not uncommon. There's nothing wrong with it, especially when your breasts are still developing. However, if you notice any breast lumps, you should have a doctor examine you just to make sure the lumps aren't tumors or cysts.
knew it/didn't know it

Q: What if my testicles are different sizes?
That's not uncommon. If the larger testicle is hard, you should have it checked by a doctor to make sure it's not a cyst, tumor, or hernia.
knew it/didn't know it

Q: What are wet dreams, and why do they happen?
Wet dreams are also known as nocturnal emissions. Starting at puberty, as a male's body goes through all sorts of changes, he's likely to have some fluid ejaculation from his penis. This usually happens at night and is often during a sexually stimulating dream—hence the term *wet dream*.
knew it/didn't know it

Q: Have I done something wrong if I have a wet dream?
Some guys feel guilty about wet dreams—maybe because it reminds them of wetting the bed or because they're dreaming about specific women. But it's really just a subconscious and natural event that doesn't necessarily mean anything.
knew it/didn't know it

Q: If the penis is withdrawn before ejaculation, can pregnancy still occur?
During extended foreplay, a small amount of preejaculatory fluid seeps from the penis. This fluid contains live sperm that can cause pregnancy. Because of this, withdrawing the penis from the vagina before ejaculation is not generally considered a safe form of birth control.
knew it/didn't know it

Q: And what exactly is foreplay?
Foreplay is the early stage of sexual "play" that gets a couple ready for intercourse. In other words, making out is foreplay.
knew it/didn't know it

Q: I've heard that a female won't get pregnant if she has sex standing up or if she has sex in a hot tub. Is that true?
A female can be jumping up and down, doing handstands, or doing cartwheels; but if she's having sex, she could get pregnant. The position doesn't matter, and neither does the environment. She can be in a hot tub, sauna, or even a waterbed—if she's having sex, she could get pregnant at any time.
knew it/didn't know it

Q: Does having sex change you physically?
For women the hymen (a membrane just inside the vagina) can break, which might hurt and cause some bleeding. If you get pregnant, there are *lots* of physical changes. For men nothing really changes physically, but either gender can pick up sexually transmitted infections—even from

having sex only once. Oh yeah, did we mention that if you're a woman, you could get pregnant? Or that if you're a man or woman, you could get HIV? We don't mean to harp, but those are pretty huge deals.

knew it/didn't know it

Q: Sex is always neat and clean in the movies—is that right?

Sex is messy—not gross necessarily, but messy. When the male ejaculates, the two-six milliliters of semen containing about 300 million sperm have to go somewhere. Plus the vagina builds up additional lubrication. You figure it out.

knew it/didn't know it

Q: Christians are so prudish. They must have lousy sex, right?

Actually, quite the opposite is the case. One national survey of 3,500 Americans ages 18 to 59 (conducted by the University of Chicago in 1994) revealed that Protestant Christian women are most likely to achieve orgasm each and every time they have vaginal intercourse. Could this be a fringe benefit of following God's plan?

Philip Elmer-Dewitt, *Time* magazine, October 17, 1994.

knew it/didn't know it

Back-to-Basics Biology

This is a cheat sheet on basic sexual biology. Use it to refresh your memory from health class. (This will not be on the test.) Feel free to circle whether you knew it or didn't.

ACCESSORY ORGANS—Sperm cells aren't capable of self-movement until ejaculation, and they're activated by seminal plasma fluid secreted by the prostate gland, ejaculatory ducts, seminal vesicles, and bulbourethral glands. These organs are important even though they can't be seen.
knew it/didn't know it

CERVIX—The opening from the vagina into the uterus, located at the far (internal) end of the vagina.
knew it/didn't know it

CLITORIS—The only organ in the human anatomy designed solely for sexual stimulation, the female clitoris is a two- to three-centimeter funnel loaded with nerve endings. It's very sensitive both to pleasure and pain.
knew it/didn't know it

CORONAL RIDGE—The bulge near the end of the penis is called the coronal ridge.
knew it/didn't know it

GLANS (OR HEAD)—If a male has been circumcised, the glans is visible at the end of the penis. If a male hasn't been circumcised, the glans is covered with loose skin called the foreskin.
knew it/didn't know it

LABIA MAJORA—The outermost ridges of the vulva designed to protect the rest of the vagina. If a female hasn't given birth, the outer lips of the labia majora probably meet at the center of her genitals.
knew it/didn't know it

OVARIES—The ovaries are female internal organs shaped like large almonds. They are located on either side of the uterus and produce some of the sex hormones that affect the menstrual cycle. But their primary function is to release one of about 400,000 eggs for reproduction 14 days before menstruation begins. The egg is either fertilized by a male's sperm and implants itself in the uterus, or it's discharged from the body with the menstrual blood flow. This process begins in puberty and continues until menopause.
knew it/didn't know it

PENIS—The penis is the external male organ for sexual intercourse and introduces sperm into the vagina. During sexual excitement, blood is temporarily trapped in the chambers of the erectile tissue in the penis, causing the penis to become enlarged, firm, and erect.
knew it/didn't know it

SCROTUM—A pouch in the male genital anatomy that holds two glands called the testes.
knew it/didn't know it

SHAFT—The cylindrical structure of the penis.
knew it/didn't know it

SPERM—Cells from a male that are capable of fertilizing a mature egg in the female reproductive system. The process of sexual arousal and ejaculation activates the otherwise immobile cells so they become self-propelled in the seminal fluid by means of a tiny tail that whips from side to side. Sperm are available more or less on demand in quantities of around 300 million cells per ejaculation. Under favorable conditions sperm live about three days after ejaculation.
knew it/didn't know it

TESTES—The testes (the primary male reproductive organ) are two small glands that move around in the scrotum and generate sperm.
knew it/didn't know it

UTERUS (WOMB)—A pear-shaped muscular organ in the female reproductive system, located between the urinary bladder and rectum and connecting through the cervix to the vagina. The lining of the uterus, the endometrium, secretes fluids that keep eggs and sperm alive and nourish fertilized eggs. If a mature egg isn't fertilized, it's flushed out with the endometrium through the vagina during menstruation.
knew it/didn't know it

> Information adapted from these resources—
>
> • *The Gift of Sex: A Christian Guide to Sexual Fulfillment* by Clifford and Joyce Penner (Word).
>
> • *Encyclopaedia Britannica CD 98,* Encyclopaedia Britannica.

URETHRA—A thin tube that carries urine from the bladder out of the body. In the male, the urethra also carries sperm from the seminal vesicles out through the penis.
knew it/didn't know it

VAGINA—A tube-shaped canal that leads from outside the body to the uterus, adapts in size to receive the penis during intercourse, and expands to accommodate a baby during delivery.
knew it/didn't know it

VULVA—The external female genitalia that surround the opening to the vagina.
knew it/didn't know it

how to help
victims of sexual abuse

What (Almost) Nobody Will Tell You about Sex can be "risky bidnez." If you start talking honestly with your friends, there's always the chance that someone will come out with something shocking. If a friend reveals sexual experiences that are troubling, frightening, even dangerous, don't freak out. Chances are, if someone chooses to trust you with a difficult story about sexual abuse, that friend won't be going off the deep end anytime soon. She's probably carried the story silently for a while, and you've given her the impression you can help. You can. You can't solve anything, but you *can* help her get the help she needs. Take a deep breath, express your sympathy, and listen intently.

If, after you hear a friend's story, you believe that a reasonable person would call it sexual abuse, chances are it is. If that's the case, the next step is help to your friend find more help than you can probably offer on your own.

If you're not sure how to do that, and if your friend doesn't believe she can get real help at home, use one or more of these resources.

- Offer to go with your friend to see a trustworthy staff member in your church or youth group. That person will probably know what to do. If you're convinced the situation is real and your staff leader seems confused or you fear the leader will sweep it under the rug, be sure you take the next steps.

- Take your friend to the head counselor or vice principal at your school—whoever seems to genuinely care about students. This person is what the law calls a *mandated reporter*. That means he is obligated by law to report sexual abuse he believes has occurred. Chances are, he will call the sheriff, police, or child protective services (or whatever it's called where you live). Law enforcement jurisdictions can be confusing, and it's easy to get lost in the system, but school personnel have probably already been through this (more often than they wish), and they'll walk you through it.

> Don't let the *mandated reporter* thing set you back. If your friend was going to solve this problem without outside help, she would have by now. So it only makes sense to call on people who can protect and defend your friend. And by the way, if you're a real expert, you're probably a mandated reporter, too.

- Get in touch with a trustworthy counselor or therapist and ask for her help. By the way, she's a mandated reporter, too. Your pastors and youth leaders are, too, though they may not know about that.

- If you go through all these channels, and you believe nothing is happening, start again at the top, express your frustration humbly, and ask for help again. You're looking for justice in a system where you probably don't feel at home. That's okay. Keep after it. They'll listen to you eventually if you don't give up.

- Tell your friends about the Girls and Boys Town hotline, 800-448-3000. Girl and Boys Town offers a full range of help, and they're very nice people.

- 800-4-A-CHILD is the number for Childhelp USA. They specialize in sexual abuse assistance. They're also very nice.

- If you fear for a friend's safety and can't seem to get the help you need locally, you can call 800-NEW-LIFE (New Life Treatment Centers' in-hospital psychiatric program) for recommendations on how to proceed. They won't try to sell you anything, and they'll give you the best information available.

2 Samuel 11:11
2 Samuel 12:24
1 Chronicles 2:21
1 Chronicles 7:23
Proverbs 5:15-20
Song of Songs (all)
Isaiah 8:3
Matthew 19:5
1 Corinthians 7:2-5

**messy multi-marital
sexual arrangements**
Genesis 16:1-16
Genesis 29:21-30
Genesis 30:1-24
Genesis 38:1-30
2 Samuel 12:11

prostitution
Genesis 38:1-30
Leviticus 19:29
Judges 16:1
Proverbs 2:11-19
Proverbs 5:1-14
Proverbs 6:20-35
Proverbs 7:1-27
Proverbs 23:26-28
Jeremiah 3:1-20
Ezekiel 16:1-42
Ezekiel 23:1-49
Hosea 3:1-3
Hosea 4:10-19
Hosea 8:9
Hosea 9:1
Nahum 3:4
1 Corinthians 6:9-10
1 Corinthians 6:12-20

rape
Deuteronomy 22:25-29
Judges 19:16-30
2 Samuel 13:1-22

seduction
Genesis 19:30-35
Genesis 38:1-30
Genesis 39:1-21
Exodus 22:16
2 Samuel 11:2-5
Proverbs 2:11-19
Proverbs 5:1-20
Proverbs 6:20-35
Proverbs 7:1-27
Proverbs 23:26-28
Jeremiah 3:1-20
Ezekiel 16:1-42
Ezekiel 23:1-49
Nahum 3:4
James 1:13-15

sex with animals
Exodus 22:19
Leviticus 18:23
Leviticus 20:15-16

sleeping around
Genesis 35:22
Exodus 22:16
Leviticus 18:6-18, 20-22
Leviticus 19:20
Leviticus 20:10-13, 19-20
Numbers 5:11-31
Numbers 25:1-3
Deuteronomy 22:22-24
Deuteronomy 27:20, 23
1 Samuel 2:22

2 Samuel 11:2-5
2 Samuel 12:11
2 Samuel 16:20-22
Proverbs 5:1-20
Proverbs 6:20-35
Proverbs 7:1-27
Proverbs 23:26-28
Jeremiah 3:1-20
Ezekiel 16:1-42
Ezekiel 23:1-49
Hosea 1:2
Hosea 2:2-15
Matthew 15:19
Matthew 19:9
Mark 7:21
John 4:16
John 8:3-11
Acts 15:20, 29
Acts 21:25
Romans 1:24-27
Romans 13:13-14
1 Corinthians 5:1-2
1 Corinthians 6:9-10
1 Corinthians 6:12-20
1 Corinthians 10:8
2 Corinthians 12:21
Galatians 5:19-21
Ephesians 5:3
Colossians 3:5
1 Thessalonians 4:3-5
Jude 1:7
Revelation 2:14
Revelation 9:21
Revelation 21:8
Revelation 22:15

wet dreams
Leviticus 15:16-17
Leviticus 22:4
Deuteronomy 23:10-11

RESOURCES FROM YOUTH SPECIALTIES

Youth Ministry Programming

Camps, Retreats, Missions, & Service Ideas
(Ideas Library)
Compassionate Kids: Practical Ways to Involve
Your Students in Mission and Service
Creative Bible Lessons from the Old Testament
Creative Bible Lessons in 1 & 2 Corinthians
Creative Bible Lessons in John: Encounters
with Jesus
Creative Bible Lessons in Romans: Faith on Fire!
Creative Bible Lessons on the Life of Christ
Creative Bible Lessons in Psalms
Creative Junior High Programs from
A to Z, Vol. 1 (A-M)
Creative Junior High Programs from
A to Z, Vol. 2 (N-Z)
Creative Meetings, Bible Lessons, &
Worship Ideas (Ideas Library)
Crowd Breakers & Mixers (Ideas Library)
Downloading the Bible Leader's Guide
Drama, Skits, & Sketches (Ideas Library)
Drama, Skits, & Sketches 2 (Ideas Library)
Dramatic Pauses
Everyday Object Lessons
Games (Ideas Library)
Games 2 (Ideas Library)
Games 3 (Ideas Library)
Good Sex: A Whole-Person Approach to
Teenage Sexuality & God
Great Fundraising Ideas for Youth Groups
More Great Fundraising Ideas for Youth Groups
Great Retreats for Youth Groups
Holiday Ideas (Ideas Library)
Hot Illustrations for Youth Talks
More Hot Illustrations for Youth Talks
Still More Hot Illustrations for Youth Talks
Ideas Library on CD-ROM
Incredible Questionnaires for Youth Ministry
Junior High Game Nights
More Junior High Game Nights
Kickstarters: 101 Ingenious Intros to Just
about Any Bible Lesson
Live the Life! Student Evangelism Training Kit
Memory Makers
The Next Level Leader's Guide
Play It! Over 150 Great Games for Youth Groups
Roaring Lambs
So What Am I Gonna Do with My Life?
Leader's Guide
Special Events (Ideas Library)
Spontaneous Melodramas
Spontaneous Melodramas 2
Student Leadership Training Manual
Student Underground: An Event Curriculum
on the Persecuted Church
Super Sketches for Youth Ministry
Talking the Walk
Videos That Teach
What Would Jesus Do? Youth Leader's Kit

Wild Truth Bible Lessons
Wild Truth Bible Lessons 2
Wild Truth Bible Lessons—Pictures of God
Wild Truth Bible Lessons—Pictures of God 2
Worship Services for Youth Groups

Professional Resources

Administration, Publicity, & Fundraising
(Ideas Library)
Dynamic Communicators Workshop for
Youth Workers
Equipped to Serve: Volunteer Youth Worker
Training Course
Help! I'm a Junior High Youth Worker!
Help! I'm a Small-Group Leader!
Help! I'm a Sunday School Teacher!
Help! I'm a Volunteer Youth Worker!
How to Expand Your Youth Ministry
How to Speak to Youth...and Keep Them Awake
at the Same Time
Junior High Ministry (Updated & Expanded)
The Ministry of Nurture: A Youth Worker's Guide
to Discipling Teenagers
Purpose-Driven Youth Ministry
Purpose-Driven Youth Ministry Training Kit
So That's Why I Keep Doing This! 52 Devotional
Stories for Youth Workers
Teaching the Bible Creatively
A Youth Ministry Crash Course
The Youth Worker's Handbook to Family Ministry

Academic Resources

Four Views of Youth Ministry & the Church
Starting Right: Thinking Theologically about
Youth Ministry

Discussion Starters

Discussion & Lesson Starters (Ideas Library)
Discussion & Lesson Starters 2 (Ideas Library)
EdgeTV
Get 'Em Talking
Keep 'Em Talking!
Good Sex: A Whole-Person Approach to Teenage
Sexuality & God
High School TalkSheets
More High School TalkSheets
High School TalkSheets from Psalms and
Proverbs
Junior High TalkSheets
More Junior High TalkSheets
Junior High TalkSheets from Psalms and Proverbs
Real Kids: Short Cuts
Real Kids: The Real Deal—on Friendship,
Loneliness, Racism, & Suicide
Real Kids: The Real Deal—on Sexual Choices,
Family Matters, & Loss
Real Kids: The Real Deal—on Stressing Out,
Addictive Behavior, Great
Comebacks, & Violence

Real Kids: Word on the Street
Unfinished Sentences: 450 Tantalizing Statement-
Starters to Get Teenagers Talking & Thinking
What If...? 450 Thought-Provoking Questions to
Get Teenagers Talking, Laughing, and Thinking
Would You Rather...? 465 Provocative Questions
to Get Teenagers Talking
Have You Ever...? 450 Intriguing Questions
Guaranteed to Get Teenagers Talking

Art Source Clip Art

Stark Raving Clip Art (print)
Youth Group Activities (print)
Clip Art Library Version 2.0 (CD-ROM)

Digital Resources

Clip Art Library Version 2.0 (CD-ROM)
Ideas Library on CD-ROM
Youth Ministry Management Tools (CD-ROM)

Videos & Video Curricula

Dynamic Communicators Workshop for
Youth Workers
EdgeTV
Equipped to Serve: Volunteer Youth Worker
Training Course
The Heart of Youth Ministry: A Morning with
Mike Yaconelli
Live the Life! Student Evangelism Training Kit
Purpose-Driven Youth Ministry Training Kit
Real Kids: Short Cuts
Real Kids: The Real Deal—on Friendship,
Loneliness, Racism, & Suicide
Real Kids: The Real Deal—on Sexual Choices,
Family Matters, & Loss
Real Kids: The Real Deal—on Stressing Out,
Addictive Behavior, Great
Comebacks, & Violence
Real Kids: Word on the Street
Student Underground: An Event Curriculum on
the Persecuted Church
Understanding Your Teenager Video Curriculum

Student Resources

Downloading the Bible: A Rough Guide to the
New Testament
Downloading the Bible: A Rough Guide to the
Old Testament
Grow For It Journal
Grow For It Journal through the Scriptures
So What Am I Gonna Do with My Life? Journaling
Workbook for Students
Spiritual Challenge Journal: The Next Level
Teen Devotional Bible
What (Almost) Nobody Will Tell You about Sex
What Would Jesus Do? Spiritual Challenge Journal
Wild Truth Journal for Junior Highers
Wild Truth Journal—Pictures of God